PRAISE FOR *UNPLUGGED*

"Mark Kaplan's story is the story of millions of patients failed by a system that medicates numbers instead of treating root causes. This book is the patient's voice the medical establishment needs to hear. Every person on a statin should read it."

—Dr. Aseem Malhotra, Cardiologist, Author of *A Statin-Free Life*

"Our genetics predict our future, our lifestyle secures it. Mark nearly died because he lived the 'healthy lifestyle' society conforms to. He was given a second shot at life armed with a new vision of what 'healthy' truly means. This book is that story. Read this to avoid repetition in your own life."

—Dr. Robert Cywes, MfD, PhD, Metabolic Surgeon

"Mark Kaplan ate a low-fat diet and avoided red meat—yet still had a heart attack at age 52. Open-minded and tenacious, this former tennis champion discovered that a healthy diet is, in fact, the very opposite of what we've been told for decades. The surprising truth is that butter, meat, and cheese need not be shunned—far from it".

—Nina Teicholz, PhD, Author of *The Big Fat Surprise*, a NYT bestseller

UNPLUGGED

How a Heart Attack at 52 Woke Me Up to the Biggest Lie in Medicine

MARK KAPLAN

UNPLUGGED: How a Heart Attack at 52 Woke Me Up to the Biggest Lie in Medicine.

This book is not intended as a substitute for medical advice. The author is not a physician. Consult your healthcare provider before making changes to your diet, medications, or health protocols.

First Edition: 2026

Published by HealthTruth Press
neo.healthtruth.ai

Cover design generated with AI assistance

Hardcover ISBN: 979-8-9964078-3-5
Paperback ISBN: 979-8-9925409-6-3
Audiobook ISBN: 979-8-9925409-7-0
Ebook ISBN: 979-8-9925409-8-7

NEO

For Sarah.

Who saved my life by telling me the truth.

For Rebecca and David.

Who will never have to learn it the hard way.

For Melanie.

Who stood by me through the darkest days.

For everyone still plugged in.

The door is open.

CONTENTS

FOREWORD

BY PHILIP OVADIA, MD, CARDIAC SURGEON

I HAVE HELD THOUSANDS OF HEARTS IN MY HANDS. I have seen the yellow, hardened plaque that chokes off blood flow. I have watched families receive news that should never have to be delivered. And time after time, the patient on the table did everything the system told them to do.

They ate a low-fat diet and minimized red meat and eggs. They went for their annual physicals. They trusted their doctors when they were told the only number that mattered was their LDL cholesterol. Many of them were on statins. Many of them were told they were "fine" or "borderline" or "managing it well." Then their hearts stopped cooperating.

Mark Kaplan's story is not an outlier. It is the rule.

Mark was the picture of what conventional medicine calls success: a former professional tennis player who had competed at Wimbledon, a fit and competitive 52-year-old who still played several times a week, a devoted husband and father who had built a good life. He had done what every responsible person is supposed to do. He had followed the guidelines. He had eaten the low-fat yogurt, the whole wheat toast, the pasta dinners. He drank the Gatorade. He avoided red meat because "they" said it was bad for his heart. And for fourteen years, seven separate blood panels had flagged one thing and one thing only: an LDL around 110. Seven times he was told to take a statin. Seven times he said no.

He was right to refuse. But the tragedy is that the system never gave him anything better to say yes to.

What Mark's story makes devastatingly clear is how narrow the medical lens has become. Our focus when it comes to preventing the leading cause of death worldwide has become overly focused on one number. We have ignored or dismissed markers that matter more. We have failed the 700,000 people in the United States that will die of heart disease this year. We have failed Mark and everyone like him.

This is not a failure of individual doctors. It is a failure of the paradigm. We have built an entire architecture of guidelines, education, and reimbursement around the idea that heart disease is primarily a cholesterol problem best managed with pharmaceuticals. The data have never supported that simplification. Seventy-five percent of patients hospitalized with heart attacks have "normal" LDL cholesterol by current standards. The real drivers—insulin resistance, chronic inflammation, metabolic dysfunction driven by a diet wildly mismatched to human physiology, and genetic vulnerabilities that load the gun—are rarely measured and almost never addressed at the root.

Mark was not unlucky. He was metabolically betrayed by the very foods and advice he was told would protect him. The carbohydrates he carb-loaded with as an athlete, the seed oils, the low-fat everything—these were not neutral. For someone carrying his genetic profile, they were actively damaging. Exercise masked the problem for decades. It did not solve it. The same pattern plays out in my operating room every week.

What makes Unplugged important is not just that Mark survived. It is that he refused to stay plugged in. He did what too few patients and too few doctors are willing to do: he questioned the narrative. He investigated. He found the physicians willing to look at the full picture instead of the convenient one. He changed what he could change—his diet, his understanding of metabolic health, his willingness to test what actually matters—and he built something from the wreckage. That is the part of his story that gives me hope.

I have written elsewhere about the need to stay off my operating table. Mark's book is a raw, personal demonstration of why that message is urgent. It is not anti-medicine. It is anti-illusion. It is a call to stop medicating numbers while the patient in front of us continues to deteriorate. It is a demand that we measure what matters and empower the patients behind those numbers to take back control of their health. To educate them on the powerful changes that they can make to what they eat and how they live.

To all the patients who have been told their cholesterol is the only thing worth worrying about: read this book. To all the doctors still practicing inside the old paradigm: read this book. To anyone who has lost someone who "did everything right": this is the story that explains why.

Mark walked off a tennis court and into the biggest lie in medicine. He fought his way back and chose to tell the truth. The least we can do is listen.

Philip Ovadia, MD Cardiac Surgeon
Founder, Ovadia Heart Health and Co-Founder, HealthTruth | Neo
Author, *Stay Off My Operating Table* and *Stay Off My Kitchen Table*
May 2026

PART ONE

INSIDE THE MATRIX

THE LIFE THAT LOOKED PERFECT.

THE HEALTH THAT LOOKED FINE.

THE SYSTEM THAT WAS QUIETLY FAILING.

CHAPTER 1

THE INVINCIBLE MAN

I HAVE BEEN AN UNDERDOG MY ENTIRE LIFE.

My parents met on a tennis court when they were fifteen years old, at a club called Jabula in Johannesburg. They got married at twenty, and we became a tennis family. All of us. Every single one of us played.

My father was the one who practiced with me. At night, when I was young, we would hit balls together under the lights while the rest of the neighborhood was settling in for dinner. I could hear the sprinklers running on the courts next to ours and the sound of the ball echoing off the fence in the dark. He played in business tennis matches during the day and golf on the weekends. He was active and competitive and he believed in me before anyone else did.

My mother watched every match I ever played. My father could not sit still. He would pace back and forth behind the fence, his nerves eating him alive, because he cared too much to watch calmly and too much to look away. But he was the one who put the racket in my hand. He was the one who hit with me when nobody else would. He was the rock.

South Africa was an outdoor life. The weather was like California. Tennis courts everywhere, golf courses in every suburb. I became a 4-handicap golfer. My father's brothers were scratch golfers and my brother played and everyone competed and everyone was driven.

That is where I got it. The drive, the hunger, the refusal to lose. It was in the family before it was ever in me.

When I was thirteen, I was middle of the pack on those courts in Johannesburg. Not the biggest kid, not the most talented, not the one anyone pointed to and said that boy is going to be something. I was just a smaller kid who had learned to fight because nobody expected anything from him.

My father gave me one thing that mattered more than talent. Optimism. The belief that every problem was an opportunity. The belief that being down was not a sentence but a starting position. And I discovered something about myself early on that would define everything that came after.

I was the most dangerous when I was losing.

When I was ahead, my mind wandered. But when my back was against the wall, everything got still. My thoughts cleared and my shots found their targets and I won more matches coming back from behind than I ever won leading from the front. Other players feared being behind. I was comfortable there. I had lived there my whole life.

At fifteen, I was nobody. At eighteen, I was top in the country. I made junior Wimbledon, and when I got to UC Irvine I did not even have a full scholarship. They gave me a few balls and a spot at the bottom of the ladder. My coach told me to go play a match against the number five guy on the team.

I beat him.

By my senior year in 1989, I had made the semifinals of the NCAA Division 1 championship. I was top five in the country with a 20-match winning streak. They voted me into the UC Irvine Hall of Fame and named me college player of the year. Arthur Ashe gave me the trophy at the US Open. Arthur Ashe. One of the greatest tennis players who ever lived, standing in front of me, handing me an award because a kid who walked on to a college team with no scholarship and no one knowing his name had become the best college player in America.

Nobody expected any of it. Least of all me.

On the professional tour, I won two tournaments quickly, got to 117 in the world, and beat top ten players. I competed at Wimbledon. A kid from Johannesburg who was middle of the pack at thirteen was now standing on the most famous tennis court in the world, the grass under his feet still wet from the morning dew, the crowd close enough to hear them breathe.

I built my business career the same way. No expectations. Fight for everything. Build it up from nothing. That was who I was.

By 52, I had everything. An amazing wife named Melanie. Three incredible children. A successful business. A house in Stamford, Connecticut. I traveled the world and played competitive tennis multiple times a week and I was the fittest person in most rooms I walked into.

I remember the trip to Lake George with my son David, right before everything changed. We rented a houseboat and it was just the two of us. Father and son. We jumped off cliffs into water so cold it took your breath away and we boated across the lake in the afternoon sun and we ate whatever we wanted and we laughed the way you laugh when nothing in the world is wrong. Everything was normal. Everything was perfect.

I would come home and play tennis at the club with my friends. Beers after the match. Sitting on the bench with a cold one in your hand, talking about your kids, the sun going down behind the courts. Life was good. I was happy. The kind of happy where you do not even think about being happy because nothing is wrong.

Sure, I was a few pounds over my playing weight. I had finished the tour at 170 and I was sitting at 195. But I did not know any different. I ate my low-fat yogurt. Had very little red meat because they said it was bad for my heart. Worried about my cholesterol because my doctor told me to. Went for my annual checkups. Did everything the system said I was supposed to do.

My dad had passed away about a year before. That was hard. But I had my family and I had my health and I had my fight.

I was invincible.

Seven blood panels over fourteen years had confirmed it. Well, not exactly. Seven blood panels had told seven different doctors that my LDL cholesterol was around 110, and seven different doctors had said the same thing: take a statin. And seven times I had said no, because I was an athlete, because I felt great, because the idea that something was wrong with me was absurd.

I did not take the statin. But I also did not know what nobody told me. That the same blood panels that flagged my cholesterol contained clues to eleven other problems, and nobody mentioned any of them. I did not know that the low-fat yogurt and the whole wheat toast and the margarine and the pasta were the exact foods that my DNA could not process without metabolic damage. I did not know that the sports drinks I had consumed for thirty years on tennis courts around the world were driving insulin resistance that was quietly building toward an event.

I did not know any of that.

I was 52 and I was happy and I was the fittest I had felt in years. I had just come back from the best trip with my son. My friend Mitch, a good tennis friend I had played with many times, called and asked if I wanted to hit some balls at Tokoneke Tennis Club in Darien.

I said yes.

I grabbed my racket and walked onto the court the same way I had walked onto thousands of courts since I was six years old. With the same optimism my father gave me. The same stubbornness that had carried me from the middle of the pack in Johannesburg to Wimbledon. The same belief that nothing could stop me.

I was invincible.

For about ten more minutes.

CHAPTER 2

OUT OF AFRICA

AFRICA IS THE CRADLE OF MANKIND.

That is not poetry. That is science. The oldest human remains ever found were discovered in Africa. Lucy. 3.2 million years old. The bones of our ancestors, preserved in the same soil where I rode my bicycle to school and played tennis until the sun went down.

I grew up on the land where humanity began. And I did not know it meant anything until a heart attack at 52 forced me to understand what we were designed to be.

Johannesburg in the 1970s was a special place to be a child. The weather was like California, warm and dry, the kind of weather that pushed you outside and kept you there until your mother called you home for dinner. But it was more than the weather. There was something primal about living in Africa, a connection to the earth that I did not have words for as a boy but I feel it now when I close my eyes and remember.

The thunderstorms in the afternoon. Massive. Rolling in like a wall of sound across the highveld, the sky going dark in minutes, and then the crack and the rain coming down so hard you could not hear your own voice. And then afterwards, the air. Clean and electric and smelling of wet earth and lightning. The doves making those soft sounds in the stillness. The sun dropping low and painting everything gold.

We walked to school and we walked to the stores and we rode our bicycles through neighborhoods where everyone knew everyone. We played until the sun went down. Tennis and golf and running in the streets with dirty knees and no shoes and no idea that the world was anything other than this.

We went on safaris. We saw the lions and the elephants and the herds of antelope moving across the plains in numbers so large they looked like a single living thing flowing across the landscape. Nature was connected to us every single day. Not as something we visited on weekends. As the air we breathed. As the ground we walked on. As the food chain we could see with our own eyes playing out in real time.

I used to watch National Geographic for hours. Even after I went to college in America, I would sit and watch the animals and how the whole system worked. The balance of everything. The lions ate the antelope. The antelope ate the grass. The grass grew from the soil. The soil was nourished by the rain. A circle. Perfect and unbroken for millions of years.

My philosophy has always been evolutionary. We are a species that evolved in nature. The fittest survive. Darwin's theory. I did not read about this in a textbook. I saw it. Growing up in Africa, I watched it play out every day. I saw the balance and the way the animals ate and the way they drank water and the way the predators kept the prey healthy by culling the weak. Everything connected. Everything in proportion. Everything working the way it was designed to work.

Years later, when I went to Kenya, I saw the Maasai. They lived in villages as a community and as a family. They ate milk and blood and meat. They were lean and fit and strong. They did not have gyms or nutritionists or food pyramids. They had the food that the land provided and the movement that survival required.

Yes, they might die of a snake bite or an infectious disease. But they were not obese. They were not insulin resistant. They were not taking statins. They were not dying of heart disease at 52.

We lived amongst the tribes in South Africa. The Zulu. The Xhosa. These were people connected to the earth in a way that modern civilization has forgotten. And something about that connection stayed inside me, even after I left. Even after forty years in America. Even after the heart attack. Because when I finally understood what had happened to my body, when I understood the root causes and the metabolic dysfunction and the mismatch between my genetics and my diet, everything pointed back to the same truth.

Nature heals. The foods we evolved to eat heal. The communities we evolved to live in heal. The movement we evolved to perform heals. And everything that had gone wrong in my body was a departure from that design.

But even in Africa, the lie had arrived.

My parents were the center of everything. My father with his optimism and his businesses. My mother with her warmth and her kitchen and her absolute certainty about what we would eat.

My mother had a set menu. Every day of the week. I could tell you what day it was by what was on the table. Monday was meatballs and spaghetti. Tuesday was schnitzels. Saturday was bagels. Sunday was Kentucky Fried Chicken.

I can still see that kitchen. I can still smell Tuesday. The schnitzels frying in the pan, the oil popping and crackling, my mother standing at the stove with a fork in her hand, the table set, the family together. Everything in its place. Everything predictable. Everything safe.

And on the counter, every morning, the yellow tub of margarine.

I can picture it right now. That soft, pale yellow spread in its plastic container. We would scrape it onto toast every morning, a thick layer, because the science said margarine was healthier than butter. Because the government guidelines said animal fat was dangerous. Because the food industry had convinced an entire generation of parents that a processed, chemically hardened vegetable oil was better for their children than the butter their grandmothers had used.

And next to the margarine, the clear bottle of oil. It said "vegetable oil" on the label. Canola oil. Safflower oil. Brilliant marketing. Vegetable oil. Vegetables are healthy, so the oil must be healthy. We knew nothing about what was actually in that bottle. We did not know it was extracted with chemical solvents and heated and deodorized and processed until it bore no resemblance to any vegetable that ever grew in the ground. We did not know that these oils would be linked to chronic inflammation decades later.

My mother fried the schnitzels in it. Tuesday's schnitzels. In canola oil from a clear bottle that said vegetable oil. It was everywhere. In the cooking, in the packages, in everything. And it had started arriving in South Africa in the 1970s, right alongside the margarine and the low-fat yogurts and the rest of the lie.

My mother was not negligent. She was the opposite. She was doing exactly what every responsible parent was told to do. Low-fat yogurts. Yoplait. I remember the containers in the fridge, the pastel colors, the word "light" on the label like a promise. Low-fat everything. Because by the 1970s, even in South Africa, the message had arrived: fat is the enemy. Eat low fat. Eat margarine. Eat grains. Follow the food pyramid.

South Africa is a country built on meat. Braais. Boerewors. Biltong. Meat is in the culture and in the soil and in our DNA. The tribes that had lived on this land for thousands of years thrived on animal protein. But by the time I was growing up, the message was creeping in. Meat is not that good for you. Go easy on the red meat. Watch the saturated fat.

Think about that. In Africa. The cradle of mankind. Where humans evolved eating meat for millions of years. The food industry convinced parents that the food their species was designed to eat was killing them. And replaced it with margarine. A product that did not exist until a chemist figured out how to harden vegetable oil in a factory.

My mother listened. Because she loved her children. Because she trusted the science. Because she had no reason to believe that the institutions telling her what to feed her family were wrong.

She fed us the lie wrapped in love. The margarine on the toast every morning. The low-fat yogurts in the fridge. The spaghetti on Monday. All of it approved. All of it endorsed. All of it slowly assembling a metabolic time bomb inside a kid who would not know it existed until he was lying in a hospital bed at 52.

I do not blame my mother. I want to say that clearly. She was a wonderful parent and she is a wonderful person. She did what every parent does. She followed the best information available and she fed her children with love and attention and consistency.

The information was the problem. Not the parent.

The dietary guidelines that reached South Africa in the 1970s were based on science that was already being questioned by the time they arrived. Ancel Keys had published his Seven Countries Study in 1958, claiming a link between dietary fat and heart disease. But he had cherry-picked his data from 22 available countries, choosing the seven that supported his hypothesis and ignoring the rest.

By the time my mother was scraping margarine onto my toast, there were scientists who knew the data was flawed. There were studies that showed no connection between saturated fat and cardiovascular disease. But those voices were drowned out by an industry that had already bet billions on the low-fat message.

The science did not drive the guidelines. The guidelines drove the market. And the market fed a generation of children food that was slowly making them sick.

I want you to understand how this happened. Not just to my mother. To every mother. To every family. To every person who has ever stood in a grocery store aisle and reached for the product with heart-healthy on the label, believing they were doing the right thing.

In 1977, the United States government told America what to eat. A senator named George McGovern chaired a committee that published the first Dietary Guidelines for Americans. The guidelines said: cut fat. Eat more grains. Follow the pyramid. And the agency that created and enforced those guidelines was the USDA.

The United States Department of Agriculture. Not the Department of Health. Not the Department of Medicine. Agriculture. An agency whose primary mandate is to promote and sell American agricultural products. Grains. Corn. Soy. Wheat. The base of the food pyramid is the product line of the agency that designed it.

That is not a conspiracy theory. That is a government org chart.

The food pyramid told Americans to eat 6 to 11 servings of bread, cereal, rice, and pasta every day. At the top of the pyramid, in the tiny triangle that said use sparingly, were fats and oils. The foods that humans had eaten for 300,000 years were put in a triangle the size of a fingernail. The foods that had been manufactured in factories for less than a century were put at the base and given 11 servings.

America listened. And America got sick.

But the guidelines were only half the lie. The other half was hiding in plain sight since 1967.

In that year, the Sugar Research Foundation, the trade group for the sugar industry, paid three Harvard scientists to publish a literature review in the New England Journal of Medicine. The review was designed to do one thing. Blame fat for heart disease and exonerate sugar. The scientists were paid the equivalent of 50,000 dollars in today's money. They published the review. It worked. For the next fifty years, the medical establishment pointed at fat while sugar quietly became the most consumed additive in the American food supply.

The payoff was not discovered until 2016. Researchers at UC San Francisco found the original correspondence, the letters, the payment records, the instructions from the sugar industry to the Harvard scientists telling them what the conclusion should be. Exposed in the Journal of the American Medical Association, Internal Medicine. Fifty years of dietary policy built on a paid conclusion. And the documents were sitting in an archive the entire time.

My mother did not know. Your mother did not know. Nobody's mother knew. They were told fat was the enemy and sugar was fine and they fed their children accordingly. Low-fat yogurt loaded with sugar. Fruit juice marketed as healthy while containing more sugar per ounce than soda. Cereal boxes with heart-healthy checkmarks that were essentially dessert in a bowl. Bread at every meal because the pyramid said so.

And then the seed oils arrived.

Soybean oil. Canola oil. Corn oil. Sunflower oil. Safflower oil. These did not exist in the human diet until the early twentieth century. They were industrial products. Lubricants. Extracted from seeds using chemical solvents, heated to extreme temperatures, deodorized to remove the rancid smell, and packaged in clear bottles with the word vegetable on the label.

In 1909, Americans consumed virtually zero seed oils. By 2010, soybean oil alone accounted for more than 7 percent of all calories consumed in America. Seed oils went from nothing to everywhere in a single century. They are in every restaurant fryer, every packaged food, every salad dressing, every cracker, every chip, every cookie. They are the invisible ingredient in the modern diet.

And the science is catching up to what our bodies already knew. Seed oils are high in omega-6 fatty acids that drive chronic inflammation when consumed in the quantities the modern diet delivers. The same inflammation that the JUPITER trial identified as a primary driver of heart disease. The same inflammation that my hs-CRP of 3.2 was screaming about while my doctor stared at my cholesterol.

The food made me inflamed. The inflammation damaged my arteries. The damaged arteries triggered a cardiac event. And the system's answer was not to fix the food. It was to prescribe a drug.

That is the connection nobody talks about. The food industry and the pharmaceutical industry are two sides of the same coin. One makes you sick. The other sells you the treatment. And neither one has any incentive to tell you the truth. Because a healthy person who eats real food and does not need a drug is a customer lost to both industries.

My mother stood at that stove in Johannesburg frying schnitzels in canola oil because the system told her it was healthy. She packed our lunches with low-fat yogurt and whole wheat sandwiches because the pyramid said so. She replaced butter with margarine because the guidelines said animal fat was dangerous. She did everything right. And everything she was told was wrong.

The information was the problem. Not the parent. Not then. Not now.

I was one of those children. Growing up in the cradle of mankind. On the same soil where Lucy's bones were found. Surrounded by tribes that thrived on meat and milk. Watching lions and elephants and the perfect balance of nature play out in front of me every day.

And eating margarine for breakfast.

We were not born statin deficient. We were born on the plains of Africa. Running and hunting and eating the food the land provided. Connected to each other and to the earth. That is what we were designed for. Everything that happened to my body was a departure from that design. And everything that healed me was a return to it.

Africa is where it started. Africa is where the truth lives.

CHAPTER 3

THE ATHLETE

WHEN I GOT TO AMERICA, I DISCOVERED A NEW RELIGION. It was called fast food, and I worshipped at its altar with the devotion of a South African kid who had never seen anything like it.

Chicken club sandwiches. Bacon cheeseburgers. Fries. McDonald's. Kentucky Fried Chicken. Not the Sunday-special KFC my mother brought home in Johannesburg. The American version. On every corner, open all hours, hot and salty and available whenever I wanted it.

I was at UC Irvine on a tennis scholarship, training every day, competing at the highest level of college tennis in America. I needed fuel. And the fuel that was available, affordable, and endorsed by every coach and sports nutritionist I encountered was the same: carbohydrates. As many as possible. As fast as possible.

Pasta before a match. Rice after practice. Bread with every meal. And Gatorade. God, the Gatorade. I can still taste it. That cold, sweet, electric-green liquid after a three-set match in the California heat, pouring it down, feeling it hit my stomach, feeling the sugar rush, believing with every cell in my body that this was exactly what my body needed. Because that is what they told us.

Sugar is energy. Carbs are fuel. Eat as much as you want. You will burn it off.

That was the gospel of sports nutrition in the 1980s and 1990s. Every college athlete heard it. Every professional athlete lived by it. The harder you trained, the more carbohydrates you consumed. The more carbohydrates you consumed, the better you performed. A simple equation. Fuel in, energy out.

Except it was wrong.

I was not overweight. That was the disguise.

I was training every day, running and hitting and competing, and my body was burning through the pasta and the rice and the Gatorade at a rate that kept me lean and fast and looking exactly like a college athlete should look. From the outside, the equation was working perfectly.

But exercise does not cancel out metabolic damage. It hides it.

You can eat a plate of pasta and burn off the calories on the court. The calorie math works. But the insulin spike does not care about the calories. Your pancreas still has to produce insulin to deal with the blood sugar surge, your liver still has to process the fructose, your cells still get bombarded with glucose. And if you do this three times a day, seven days a week, for years, the machinery starts to wear.

I did not know any of this. Nobody did. Or if they did, they were not telling college tennis players.

My second year at UC Irvine, all the seniors had left and the top spots were up for grabs. We had challenge matches and tournaments and I won the Rolex Invitational. And then I entered the NCAA Division 1 championship as a sophomore.

I made it to the semifinals. Singles and doubles. A walked-on player with no expectations was now two matches away from the national title. I lost in the semifinal to Andrew Burrow from the University of Miami. He was a senior and I was a sophomore. He went on to win the whole thing. I went back to Irvine knowing I belonged.

By my senior year, I was a top five player in the nation with a 20-match winning streak. UC Irvine was ranked outside the top 40 when I walked on as a freshman in 1986. By 1989, we were ranked number three in the country.

And in my last match as a UC Irvine player, we played UCLA. Ranked number one in the country. The match was tied. It came down to my court. My match. My point.

I won it in three sets.

A kid who walked on with no scholarship in 1986 to a team nobody knew just beat the number one team in the country in his last match, with the deciding point. That is how my college career ended. Not with a whimper. With a win over number one.

They voted me college player of the year. Athlete of the year. Inducted me into the UC Irvine Hall of Fame. All in my senior year, 1989. And Arthur Ashe gave me the trophy at the US Open.

I need you to understand what that moment meant. Arthur Ashe. One of the greatest tennis players in history. A man who broke barriers, who stood for integrity and courage and doing things the right way. And he was standing in front of me at the US Open, handing me a trophy, because a kid from Johannesburg who walked on to a college team with no scholarship and no one knowing his name had become the best college player in America.

Here is the part I did not know that day.

Arthur Ashe had a heart attack in 1979. At 36 years old. While holding a tennis clinic. Despite being at peak physical fitness. His heart disease was largely hereditary. He underwent two major bypass surgeries, and during one of them he received a blood transfusion that gave him HIV. He died in 1993 of AIDS-related pneumonia. He was 49 years old.

A heart attack at 36. On a tennis court. Despite peak physical fitness. Driven by a genetic condition involving high Lp(a). Hereditary.

I had a heart attack at 52. On a tennis court. Despite peak physical fitness. High Lp(a). Hereditary.

Arthur Ashe had Lp(a). I have Lp(a). The same genetic marker. The same inherited particle that promotes plaque buildup in arteries regardless of how fit you are, how clean you eat, how hard you train. He did not know he had it because back then nobody tested for it. He was carb-loading the same way I was carb-loading. Pasta, sports drinks, the performance diet. Fueling his tennis and fueling his disease at the same time. And he had no idea what it was doing to him.

Neither did I.

The man who handed me that trophy was living the same story I would live. Two tennis players with the same genetic marker, eating the same diet, trusting the same system, on the same path toward the same disease.

He did not make it. Heart attack at 36. Quadruple bypass. A second surgery. HIV from a blood transfusion. Dead at 49.

I made it. I was the lucky one. My widow maker did not close completely. I got to the hospital in time. The stent went in, and six years later I am still here, still playing tennis, still alive. Arthur Ashe was not lucky. The system failed him at 36 the same way it failed me at 52. The only difference is I survived long enough to find the truth.

And my son David knows at 16.

Three lives. Arthur Ashe. Mark Kaplan. David Kaplan. The same genetics. The same Lp(a). The same loaded gun. Arthur did not know. He died at 49. I did not know. I almost died at 52. David knows. He was tested at 15. He eats for his genetics. His markers are optimal. He will never have a heart attack on a tennis court wondering why the fittest person in the room is the one who fell.

That is why I built HealthTruth | Neo. For Arthur. For me. For David. For every athlete who is told they are healthy because they are fit while the disease builds silently inside them. Because the information that could have saved Arthur Ashe's life in 1979 now exists. It costs $30. And nobody is ordering it.

I went from the bottom of the ladder to a trophy from Arthur Ashe. That is who I was. That is the underdog story that defined everything. And it is the same stubbornness that would save my life thirty years later when a cardiologist told me I could die on Monday and I chose to fight.

All of that from a kid who walked on with a few balls and no expectations.

The professional tour was more of the same. Magnified.

My first real tournament win came at the California Open. It was only my second ATP event ever, and I almost lost in the first round of qualifying. Almost went home before the tournament even started. But I won that match, then the next, then the next, through qualifying and through the main draw, all the way to the final.

In the final I played my nemesis, a guy from Pepperdine who had beaten me badly in every college match. He had won the NCAAs that year. By every measure, he was supposed to win. But something happened to me in that match that I cannot explain except to say it felt like an out-of-body experience. I stayed back and I did not force anything and I did not make the errors that had cost me every other time. I just played. At a level I had never reached before. An unconscious level. The kind of tennis where your body knows what to do and your mind gets out of the way.

I beat him 6-4, 6-4.

Two months later, I won the Cape Town Challenger. Back in South Africa. Another title. The momentum was building.

Then came Queen's Club. The week before Wimbledon. The warm-up tournament where the best grass court players in the world prepare for the biggest stage in tennis. I qualified, won three matches just to get into the main draw, and won my first round.

And in the second round, I played Pete Sampras.

Pete Sampras. On the centre court of Queen's Club. In front of a full crowd that smelled like freshly cut grass and expensive cologne. I had won four matches in a week to be standing on that court, and across the net was the best player in the world. I was not supposed to be there. But the underdog from Johannesburg who was middle of the pack at thirteen was now sharing a court with Sampras. That was the moment I knew.

I have arrived.

Two weeks later, Wimbledon. I walked through those gates and I could not believe where I was. The hallowed grass courts. The grounds I had watched on television since I was a boy in Johannesburg, sitting on the floor of our living room watching McEnroe and Borg and Connors play on these same courts. And now I was being handed a pass and told which court was mine.

Court 13.

My father was there. My mother was there. Walking the grounds with strawberries and cream, wearing their best clothes, trying not to look too proud and failing completely. The white clothing, the tradition, the weight of history in every blade of grass. My parents watching their son from Johannesburg live the dream they had helped him build since he was six years old hitting balls under the lights at Jabula.

I played Jim Courier in the first round. One of the top players in the world. I was nervous and the moment was bigger than any match I had played. But I was there. On a court I had dreamed about my entire life.

The results kept coming. I was ranked number 117 ATP player in the world. I made the finals of the US Clay Courts. I beat many former top ten players in the world, including Patrick Rafter, a former world number one, Tim Henman, Malivai Washington, and Mark Philippoussis. The underdog from Johannesburg was taking them down.

And I was carb-loading before every match. Energy bars, sports drinks, pasta dinners. The performance diet that every tournament, every trainer, every sports medicine doctor endorsed. Refined carbohydrates pushed into my body at the highest rate of my life, day after day, tournament after tournament, year after year.

I was burning through it on the court. I was performing. I was winning. And the scoreboard said everything was fine.

But the scoreboard does not measure insulin resistance. The scoreboard does not measure chronic inflammation. The scoreboard does not measure thyroid function or arterial damage or the slow, silent accumulation of metabolic dysfunction that the carbohydrates were driving. My body was keeping two sets of books. The public set said world-class athlete, peak performance, no problems. The private set said insulin climbing, inflammation building, thyroid flagging, arteries hardening.

And nobody audited the private set because nobody knew it existed.

Here is what I wish someone had told me when I was twenty years old.

You carry APOE e3/e4. That gene means your body processes dietary carbohydrates and fats differently than most people. The pasta and bread and Gatorade that your teammates can eat without consequence are causing metabolic damage in your body that will not show up for thirty years.

You carry 9p21 GG. That gene means your arteries are more vulnerable to damage from inflammation. The seed oils in the fast food you eat every day and the chronic insulin spikes from the carbohydrate loading are creating exactly the conditions that your genetics cannot handle.

The markers that would have saved Arthur Ashe are available today. They cost less than a tennis lesson. Nobody is ordering them.

Eat meat. Eat eggs. Eat fish. Eat the foods your great-grandmother in South Africa would have recognized. Stop eating the foods that come in packages with health claims on the label.

Nobody said any of that. Not my coaches, not the team doctor, not the sports nutritionist, not the tour physicians, not anyone. Because in the 1980s and 1990s, saying that carbohydrates might be harmful to an athlete was like saying gravity might not be real.

It was unthinkable. The entire edifice of sports nutrition was built on the assumption that carbohydrates were the optimal fuel. Questioning it was not just wrong. It was heretical.

So I did not question it. I ate what they told me to eat and I performed at the highest level and I felt great. And every plate of pasta, every bottle of Gatorade, every chicken club sandwich was loading the gun that would fire twenty-five years later on a tennis court in Darien, Connecticut.

I was the fittest person in every room I walked into. And I was slowly destroying myself with the food I ate to stay that way.

CHAPTER 4

THE GOOD LIFE

MY FATHER WAS THE MOST IMPORTANT PERSON IN MY LIFE.

I never heard him complain. Not once in my entire life. I never heard him say something negative about anyone or anything. He was the most optimistic, positive person I have ever known, and he lit up every room he walked into. Every conversation with him left you feeling better than you did before it started. He had a way of making you believe that whatever problem you were facing was smaller than you thought and that you were bigger than you knew.

On his tombstone, it says: Life is made up of moments and memories.

That is how he lived. Every single day. He traveled a lot and he worked a lot. He built businesses in South Africa and later in America, and he was always moving, always building, always looking for the next opportunity. But every time we were together, it was a special time. He was present. Not checking his watch, not thinking about the next meeting, not distracted by the noise of his own ambition. Just there. Making the moment count. Making you feel like you were the only person in the world.

When I left South Africa at eighteen to go to college in California, my mother knew I was not coming back. And my father, without hesitation, made the decision to immigrate. The whole family. To America. Because his son was there and that was reason enough. He helped me financially. I had a half scholarship my first year and he covered the rest. After my first year I earned a full scholarship, and he helped me through my BA in Economics and then my MBA, both at UC Irvine. I would not be in America today without my father.

But it was not the money. It was the attitude. My father gave me the belief that I could never lose. Not in a naive way. In a deep, unshakable way that settled into my bones and stayed there. On the tennis court, I never felt like I was down and I never felt like I was going to lose, because I was raised by a man who never saw the glass as half empty. He always saw that there was some water in the glass. And that is how I view life. That is how I have always viewed life.

We worked together for thirteen years. Side by side. Building companies and traveling the world. He taught me business the way he had taught me life. By doing it. By showing me what it looked like when a man with relentless optimism met a problem that seemed impossible and refused to back down.

My mother was the same. Both of my parents were extraordinary. I was lucky and I knew I was lucky. Not everyone gets to grow up watching two people who love each other, love their children, and love the work they do. I had that.

And so by the time I was in my forties, the blueprint was working. I had everything my father had shown me was possible.

An amazing wife. Melanie. I met her at a wedding in San Diego. I was thirty. Finished the tour. Finished my MBA. She was living in Johannesburg. We were introduced at someone else's wedding, a blind get-together that neither of us had planned.

I told her not to fly back to South Africa. Stay. We drove up to Santa Barbara with the windows down and the Pacific on our left, and then back to New York, and before she left to go home I proposed.

Two and a half weeks. That is how long I knew her before I asked her to spend the rest of her life with me.

That is who I was. Spontaneous. Certain. The same instinct that made me dangerous on a tennis court when I was down two sets. I did not overthink and I did not plan. I saw what I wanted and I went after it. And I knew I loved this woman the way I knew I could beat a player ranked above me. Something in my gut said yes.

So I said yes.

She said yes too.

Melanie became the person who grounded me. Who raised our three children while I traveled and competed and built things. Who made the house in Stamford feel like a home. Three incredible kids. Sarah. Rebecca. David. Each one different, each one carrying some piece of me and some piece of Melanie and becoming something entirely their own. A career that was working. A body that was working. A life that looked from the outside like a man who had everything figured out.

I ate what the system told me to eat.

Every morning was the same. Low-fat yogurt. Whole wheat toast. Maybe some fruit. A glass of orange juice. The breakfast that every doctor, every nutritionist, every government guideline said was the foundation of a heart-healthy diet.

I avoided red meat because they said it was bad for my heart. I used margarine instead of butter because they said butter clogged your arteries. I ate pasta for dinner because complex carbohydrates were supposed to be the foundation of the food pyramid. I drank Gatorade after tennis because sports drinks replaced electrolytes and kept you hydrated and performing.

I did this for thirty years.

Not because I was lazy. Not because I did not care about my health. Because I trusted the science. The same way I trusted my doctors when they checked my blood panels. The same way I trusted my cardiologist when he said the only number that mattered was cholesterol. I was a responsible person making responsible choices based on the best information available.

Except the information was wrong. The margarine was full of trans fats. The low-fat yogurt was loaded with sugar. The whole wheat toast was spiking my insulin. The Gatorade was pure refined carbohydrate. The pasta was driving blood sugar and insulin to levels my APOE e4 genotype could not process.

Every morning I sat at my kitchen table eating a meal that was slowly killing me. And I felt virtuous doing it. I felt healthy. I was checking the boxes, doing the right thing, following the plan.

My annual checkups confirmed it. My doctor would look at my blood panel, flag the LDL, recommend a statin. I would say no. Everything else looked fine. See you next year. The system told me I was healthy, and I believed it, because I had never had a reason not to.

We had a good life. I want to be clear about that. This is not a story about a man who was miserable before the heart attack. This is a story about a man who was happy.

Playing tennis with my friends at the club. Beers afterward, sitting on the bench with the sun going down, talking about our kids and our businesses and our plans. Traveling with Melanie. Watching Sarah and Rebecca and David grow up. Going to their games. Driving them to school. The ordinary, beautiful, unremarkable days that you do not appreciate until they are gone.

I was a few pounds over my playing weight. But I was 52. Everyone puts on a little weight. I was still active, still competitive, still the guy who walked into a room and people said that guy is in great shape for his age.

I did not know what was building inside me. Nobody did. Because nobody looked.

Then my father had a stroke.

I was in Las Vegas for a business meeting. I came out of the hotel into the dry desert heat and my phone rang. My sister.

Dad is in the hospital. It is pretty bad. He has had a stroke.

I stood there on the sidewalk in Las Vegas with the noise of the strip behind me and my world shifted.

What I did not know then, but I know now, is that my father had been dealing with his own heart problems for years. He had an irregular heartbeat, the kind that makes your heart flutter and skip and never quite settle into the rhythm it is supposed to have. They put him on Coumadin, a blood thinner, to prevent the clots that an irregular heart can produce. He never had a CAC scan. Nobody ever checked for calcium building in his arteries. Nobody looked at his genetics. Nobody tested the root causes. The system managed his irregular heartbeat with a blood thinner and called it handled.

Then he was between medications. A gap. A window where the blood thinner was not in his system. And a clot formed and the clot reached his brain.

That is what caused the stroke. Not a random event. Not bad luck. A system that managed one symptom with one drug and never looked at the root cause. The same system that would fail me two years later on a tennis court in Connecticut.

I got to the airport and I got on the plane. Window seat. Five and a half hours from Las Vegas to New York. I put my head against the window and I broke down.

This was my hero. The man who taught me to be optimistic. The man who built businesses with me for thirteen years. The man who played tennis with me when I was six years old under the lights at Jabula and set me on a path that led to Wimbledon. He was in a hospital bed and my sister's voice had told me everything I needed to know.

It was the longest flight of my life. Five and a half hours with my forehead pressed against cold glass. Crying. Trying not to let the person in the next seat see. Failing. Not caring.

I saw him in the hospital. He lasted ten days.

Ten days. The most important person in my life. The blueprint. The role model. The man whose optimism I had carried like a torch from Johannesburg to California to Connecticut. Gone.

Eight months later, I was on a tennis court in Darien.

Eight months. That is all the time that separated my father's death from my heart attack. I do not know if the stress contributed. I do not know if the grief did something to my body that the blood panels could not measure. I know that my calcium score was high, which means the disease had been building for years, long before the stroke, long before the grief.

But I also know this. I lost my father eight months before I nearly became him.

Not from the same disease. Not in the same way. But in the same system. The same system that watched his health without seeing the root causes. The same system that would watch mine and miss every marker while obsessing over one.

The good life was real. The happiness was real. The family and the tennis and the breakfasts and the checkups and the feeling that everything was fine. All of it was real. But underneath it, something was building. In my arteries and in my metabolism and in my thyroid and in my insulin levels and in the genetics that nobody thought to test. The gun was loading. One chamber at a time. Year after year. Plate of pasta after plate of pasta. Low-fat yogurt after low-fat yogurt. Flagged blood panel after flagged blood panel.

I did not know any of that. I only knew that I had lost my father and that the world felt different now. Smaller. More fragile.

And then one morning, Mitch asked me to play tennis.

And I said yes.

CHAPTER 5

NORMAL CHOLESTEROL

I WANT TO TELL YOU ABOUT THE SEVEN BLOOD PANELS THAT ALMOST KILLED ME.

Over the course of fourteen years, from age 39 to 52, I had seven complete blood panels. Seven times a doctor looked at my blood. Seven times a lab printed out a report with my numbers on it. Seven times a medical professional reviewed those numbers and told me what to do.

Every single panel flagged one thing. LDL cholesterol. High.

I put that word in quotes for a reason. My LDL was around 110 for most of my life. One hundred and ten. That is not high by any reasonable standard. But the guidelines said it should be lower, and every doctor I saw for fourteen years looked at 110 and said the same two words.

Take a statin.

For a number of 110. I said no. Seven times. Because I was an athlete, because I felt great, because the guy looking back at me in the mirror did not look like someone with a heart problem. I was wrong about that last part. But the doctors were wrong about something much bigger.

They were watching one number. They missed eleven.

Let me walk you through what was sitting in those blood panels. Right there. On the same pages. In the same lab reports that my doctors were holding in their hands when they told me the only thing wrong with me was cholesterol.

My TSH was flagged high.

TSH is thyroid stimulating hormone. When it is high, it means your thyroid is underperforming, that your brain is sending louder and louder signals to your thyroid saying wake up, work harder, I need more. It is one of the most basic markers in medicine, and my TSH was flagged high in four of my seven panels. Four out of seven. Over fourteen years.

Not one doctor mentioned it.

Not one doctor referred me to an endocrinologist. Not one doctor said, hey Mark, your thyroid has been struggling for years and that can increase your cardiovascular risk significantly. Dr. Broda Barnes published research in 1976 connecting thyroid dysfunction to heart disease. 1976. Almost fifty years before my heart attack. The science was there. It was just buried. Because there is no blockbuster drug for thyroid optimization. There is no twenty billion dollar market in checking TSH.

Four flags. Fourteen years. Zero conversations.

Here is what else was never ordered.

Fasting insulin. The earliest marker of metabolic dysfunction. It goes wrong ten to fifteen years before your blood sugar ever moves. A test that has existed since 1965 and costs about thirty dollars. Available at any lab in the country.

Joseph Kraft ran this test on 14,384 patients in 1975 and found that 75 percent of people with normal blood sugar already had pathological insulin patterns. Three quarters. Forty years before my heart attack, the science showed that fasting insulin catches disease that blood sugar misses.

My doctor never ordered it. Not once. If he had, he would have found a man whose pancreas was working almost twice as hard as it should, a man with insulin resistance forming, a man with metabolic dysfunction quietly building toward a cardiac event. He would have seen it years before the ambulance arrived.

But there is no pill to prescribe when fasting insulin comes back high. There is no Pfizer product for early insulin resistance. So the test does not get ordered.

Then there was hs-CRP, a measure of systemic inflammation and one of the strongest independent predictors of cardiovascular events. Never ordered. Homocysteine, an amino acid that at elevated levels damages the lining of blood vessels and increases clotting risk. Never ordered. Lp(a), a genetic lipoprotein that is the single strongest inherited risk factor for cardiovascular disease, something you either have or you do not, something that does not respond to diet or exercise because it is entirely genetic. Never ordered.

APOE genotype. A hundred dollar genetic test that tells you how your body processes fat and cholesterol. I carry APOE e3/e4, which means my body handles dietary fat differently than 75 percent of the population. The diet I had been eating for thirty years, the pasta and the bread and the Gatorade and the low-fat everything, was the exact diet my genotype cannot process without metabolic damage. One hundred dollars. Never tested.

And then there is the test that could have shown the disease itself. Not a marker. Not a predictor. The actual disease.

A coronary artery calcium scan. A CAC score. A simple, low-dose CT scan that takes ten minutes and costs about a hundred dollars. It shows you how much calcium has built up in your coronary arteries. Calcium means plaque. Plaque means heart disease is already there.

When I finally got one, after my heart attack, my score was over 1000.

I never knew my calcium score before that day. Not once in fourteen years of checkups did anyone order a scan. I only found out after I was already lying in a hospital bed with a stent in my widow maker artery. A score of 1000 means the disease had been building in my arteries for decades. Not years. Decades. A scan in my forties would have shown plaque forming. A scan in my early fifties would have been a five-alarm fire. It would have triggered every investigation that my cardiologist never ran and caught the disease ten, maybe twenty years before it stopped my heart on a tennis court.

But my doctor never ordered it. And here is the dirty secret about why. Statins raise calcium scores. The drug that is supposed to protect your heart actually increases the calcium in your arteries. If a cardiologist puts you on a statin and then orders a calcium scan six months later and the score goes up, the patient asks questions the doctor does not want to answer.

So they do not order the scan. A hundred dollar test that could have caught the disease building in my arteries for twenty years. Never ordered. Because the result might contradict the treatment.

So let me add this up.

Seven blood panels. Fourteen years. One doctor after another looking at the same reports. What they tested: total cholesterol and LDL. What they missed: TSH flagged four times and ignored, fasting insulin, hs-CRP, homocysteine, Lp(a), APOE genotype, 9p21 genotype, HOMA-IR, triglyceride-to-HDL ratio, vitamin D, and a hundred dollar calcium scan that would have shown the disease building in my arteries for decades.

They tested two markers. They missed eleven.

And the two they tested are among the weakest predictors of heart disease in the medical literature. The Women's Health Study followed 27,939 women for twenty years and published in JAMA Cardiology. The results are devastating. Diabetes increases your risk by 10 times. Metabolic syndrome by 6 times. Obesity by nearly 4 times. Hypertension by 3.5 times. Smoking by 3.5 times.

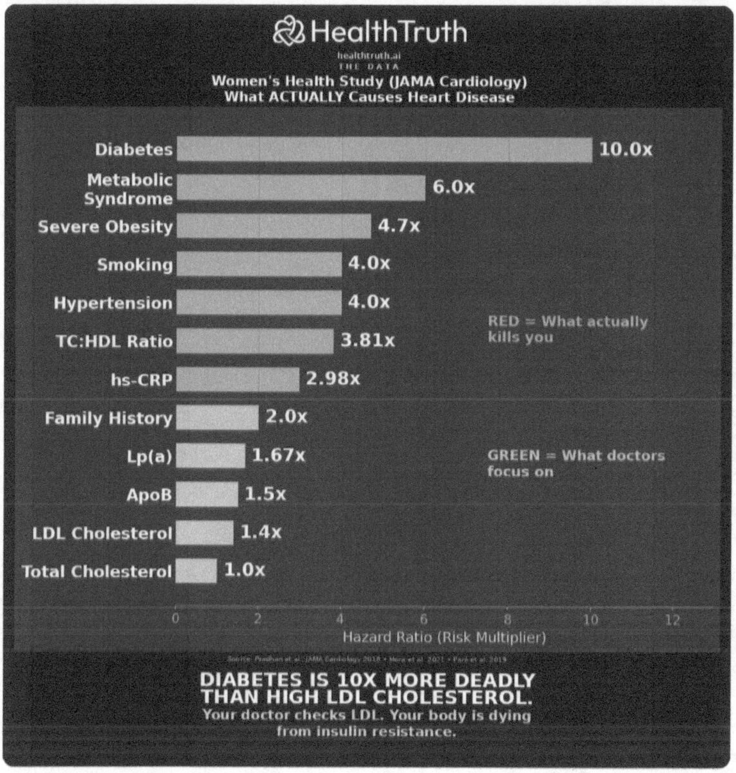

Women's Health Study (Pradhan et al., JAMA Cardiology, 2018). 27,939 women followed for 20 years. Hazard ratios for heart disease.

LDL cholesterol. 1.4 times.

The weakest predictor on the list. The thing they spent fourteen years telling me to medicate was a 1.4 times risk factor while the things they never tested were four, six, ten times more dangerous.

And here is the number that should stop you cold. Sachdeva published a study in the American Heart Journal in 2009, looking at 136,905 patients hospitalized with heart attacks. Seventy-five percent of them had LDL cholesterol levels that were considered normal by current guidelines.

Normal cholesterol. Three quarters of the people in that study had a heart attack with normal cholesterol. The number my doctors spent fourteen years trying to lower was in range for 75 percent of the people who actually had heart attacks.

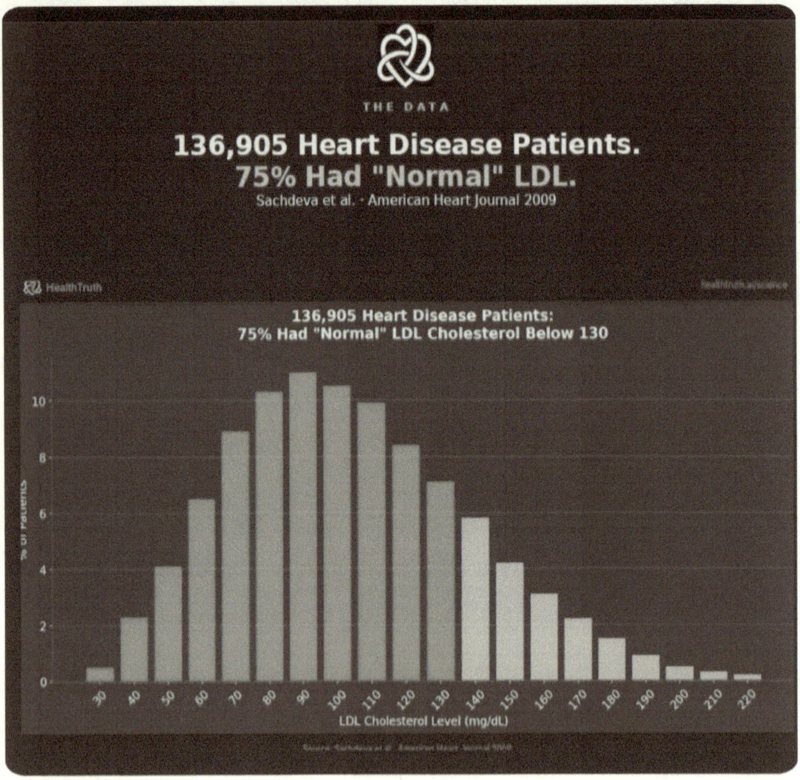

Sachdeva A et al., Lipid levels in patients hospitalized with coronary artery disease. American Heart Journal, 2009.

I need to tell you something about cholesterol that your doctor was never taught.

Your body makes cholesterol. On purpose. Every single day. Your liver produces approximately 80 percent of the cholesterol in your blood. You could eat zero cholesterol, not a single egg, not a bite of steak, not a gram of butter, and your liver would still manufacture cholesterol because your body cannot survive without it.

Every cell membrane in your body is built with cholesterol. Without it, your cells would collapse. Your brain is 25 percent cholesterol by weight, the most cholesterol-dense organ you have. It uses cholesterol to form synaptic connections, to transmit signals between neurons, to create the neurotransmitters that regulate your mood and your memory and your ability to think. Your body uses cholesterol to produce vitamin D, testosterone, estrogen, cortisol, and every other steroid hormone. It uses cholesterol to produce bile acids that digest the food you eat. It uses cholesterol to repair damaged tissue.

Cholesterol is not a poison. Cholesterol is a building material. Your body manufactures it the same way a construction company manufactures concrete. It makes it because it needs it. And when a drug forces that production down to levels the body was never designed to sustain, the body does not thank you. The body breaks.

That is what happened to me on 80 milligrams of Lipitor. My cholesterol was crushed to 40 and my brain stopped working. Not because I was aging. Because the organ that needs cholesterol more than any other organ in my body was being starved of it.

But how did we get here? How did a molecule that your body manufactures on purpose become the villain of modern medicine?

I told you about Ancel Keys in an earlier chapter. The Seven Countries Study. The 22 countries he had access to and the seven he chose because they supported his hypothesis. My mother was scraping margarine onto my toast because of that study. But cherry-picking the data was just the beginning. What happened next was worse.

In 1961, the American Heart Association issued its first dietary guidelines recommending Americans reduce saturated fat intake. Based on a study that had excluded fifteen countries worth of data.

Then something worse happened. A study was conducted that should have settled the debate forever. And they buried it.

The Minnesota Coronary Experiment ran from 1968 to 1973. It was one of the most rigorous dietary trials ever designed. Over 9,000 patients in state mental hospitals and a nursing home. They replaced saturated fat with vegetable oil, exactly what the guidelines recommended. They lowered cholesterol. The intervention worked on the number.

And then more people died.

For every 30 points they lowered cholesterol, the risk of death increased by 22 percent. The group that followed the heart-healthy diet, the group that did exactly what the government told them to do, had worse outcomes. Lower cholesterol. Higher death.

The lead researcher was Ancel Keys himself. He was a co-investigator on this study. The study that disproved his own hypothesis.

They did not publish the results. Not the full results. A partial publication appeared in 1989, sixteen years after the trial ended, and it omitted the mortality data. The complete dataset was not recovered until 2016 when researchers found the original records in a basement. Boxes of data from a landmark trial, sitting in a basement for decades because the results contradicted the dietary guidelines that had already been set in stone.

2016. I had my heart attack in 2020. The data proving that lowering cholesterol increased death had been sitting in a basement for over forty years while 92 million Americans took a drug to lower their cholesterol.

The Framingham Heart Study tells a similar story. Framingham is the longest-running cardiovascular study in history, following residents of a Massachusetts town since 1948. It is the study that the cholesterol hypothesis was supposed to be built on.

But the directors of the Framingham Study said something that most doctors have never read. In a 1992 editorial, they wrote that after the age of 50, there is no increased overall mortality with either high or low cholesterol. They found that for every one percent drop in cholesterol, there was an 11 percent increase in coronary and total mortality. The lower the cholesterol went, the higher the risk of dying.

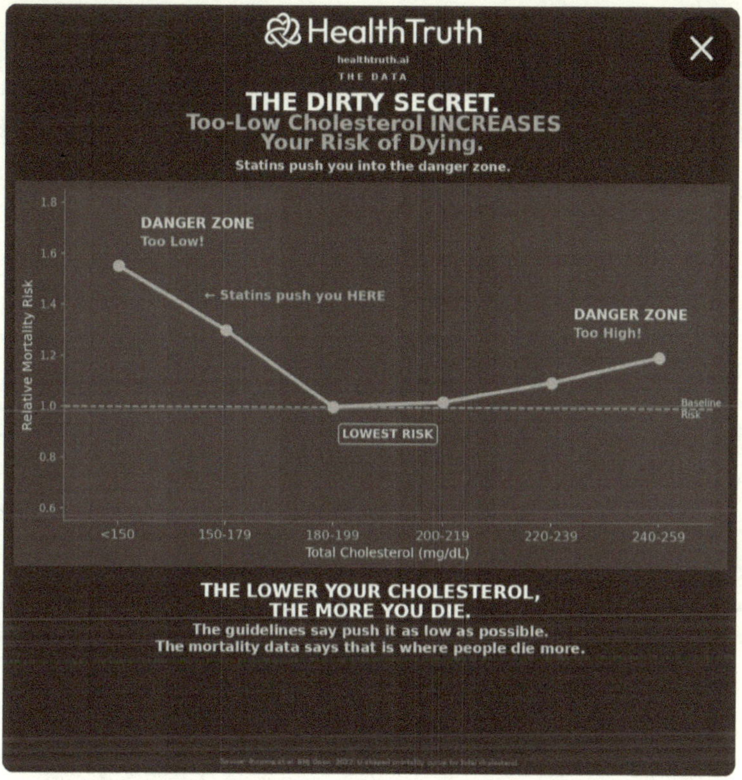

Buurma et al, BMJ Open, 2022. U-shaped mortality curve for total cholesterol.

The directors of the study that is supposed to prove cholesterol kills you published data showing the opposite. And the guidelines did not change.

In 1977, the McGovern Committee set the United States Dietary Guidelines. They told America to cut fat. Eat more grains. Follow the food pyramid. The nation listened. Fat consumption went down. Carbohydrate consumption went up. And over the next forty years, obesity tripled. Type 2 diabetes exploded. Heart disease remained the number one killer.

America followed the guidelines. The guidelines made America sick.

And here is what connects all of this back to the seven blood panels my doctors held in their hands for fourteen years. The entire architecture of cardiovascular medicine, the guidelines, the drug recommendations, the standard of care, the insurance reimbursement codes, the medical school curriculum, is built on a hypothesis that was cherry-picked from the start, contradicted by its own trials, and buried when the data did not cooperate.

My doctors were not bad people. They were trained inside a system that was built on a lie. They watched my LDL because that is what they were taught to watch. They recommended a statin because that is what the guidelines told them to recommend. They never tested my fasting insulin or my thyroid or my inflammation because the system never told them those markers mattered.

The cholesterol hypothesis is not a scientific consensus. It is an institutional consensus. Built on selected data, sustained by pharmaceutical revenue, and protected by a medical establishment that has staked fifty years of credibility on a number that the evidence says is the weakest predictor on the list.

I was one of those people. My cholesterol was not the problem. It was never the problem. My cholesterol was a distraction, a shiny number that was easy to measure, easy to medicate, and easy to bill for. While the real causes sat there quietly in my body for over a decade. The insulin resistance. The inflammation. The thyroid dysfunction. The genetic mismatches. Untested. Undetected. Unmentioned.

This is not a conspiracy theory. This is math.

A standard lipid panel costs about twenty-five dollars and takes five minutes to review. It generates a statin prescription that costs two hundred to four hundred dollars per year and requires follow-up visits every three to six months for the rest of your life.

A comprehensive metabolic and genetic workup costs three hundred to five hundred dollars and might reveal that the patient does not need a drug at all. That the solution is dietary. That the solution is a fifteen dollar bottle of magnesium. That the solution is addressing a thyroid issue that was hiding in plain sight for fourteen years.

One path generates recurring revenue for decades. The other generates a one-time intervention that fixes the problem.

The system is not broken by accident. It is broken by design.

And my seven blood panels are the evidence.

PART TWO

THE CRASH

THE MOMENT THE MATRIX BREAKS.
THE SYSTEM REVEALS ITSELF.
EVERYTHING CHANGES.

CHAPTER 6

TENNIS COURT TO OPERATING TABLE

ONE STROKE.

That is all it took. One forehand. Maybe a backhand. I do not even remember which. Mitch and I had not warmed up much, we were just getting into it, singles the way we always played, and after one stroke I knew something was wrong.

I could not breathe.

Not the kind of breathless you get after a long rally. Not the kind where you bend over and put your hands on your knees and recover in thirty seconds. This was different. This was my body refusing to give me air. Like someone had put a hand over my mouth and nose and was not letting go.

I stopped playing and sat down on the bench next to the court. The sun was out. The courts were quiet. I waited for it to pass.

It did not pass.

There was a feeling in my stomach. Not pain exactly. More like acid reflux. A pressure, something sitting there that should not have been there. And I still could not catch my breath. I had played thousands of matches in my life, on courts all over the world, and I had never felt anything like this.

I did what every person my age does when something does not feel right. I pulled out my phone, sat on the bench at Tokoneke Tennis Club in Darien, Connecticut, and Googled my symptoms.

Shortness of breath. Acid reflux. Can't catch breath.

The results came back, and somewhere in those results it mentioned the heart. But this was a unique feeling. I had had sore stomachs and headaches and flu and aches and pains. Every normal thing that happens to a body over 52 years. But this was different. This was a shortness of breath that I had never experienced before. Something was wrong with my body and I knew it.

I just did not know what.

I did not panic. Not yet. I had things to do. My daughter Rebecca needed to be picked up from soccer practice. That is how normal this day was supposed to be. Tennis with Mitch. Pick up Rebecca. Go home. Have dinner. Normal.

So I drove to the soccer field, picked her up, drove her home. Still not breathing right, still feeling that pressure, and I did not say a word to her in the car. You do not want to cause alarm when you are not really sure what is going on. You are her father and you are supposed to be the strong one. So you drive and you stay quiet and you tell yourself it is probably nothing.

Besides, you think, it cannot be a heart attack. Heart attacks are when you hold your chest and drop to the ground. I did not have that. I was still standing, still driving, still functioning. So it cannot be a heart attack. That is what you tell yourself because the alternative is too terrifying to say out loud while your daughter is in the back seat.

I dropped her at the house and then I drove to the Tully Center, a walk-in clinic near our home. Not an ER. A walking clinic. I walked in and I waited, because that is what you do at a walk-in clinic. You wait. I sat there in a plastic chair with fluorescent lights humming above me and other people waiting for other things, coughs and sprains and flu symptoms, and finally I said to the nurse at the desk: look, something is not right. Can you take a look at me?

They brought me in and put the EKG wires on me, all these wires attached to my chest, cold adhesive pads pressed against my skin. It took a few minutes. And then the nurse looked at the screen and her expression changed. The waves were not right. Something had happened.

She said: you need to go to the hospital. There is something that does not look right.

That is when I got concerned. Not panicked. Concerned. There is a difference. Panic shuts you down. Concern keeps you moving. And I needed to keep moving.

I grabbed the piece of paper with the EKG results and I drove myself to Stamford Hospital, about two miles away. And while I was driving, gripping the steering wheel with one hand and the EKG printout folded on the passenger seat beside me, it was hard to fathom that this was actually happening. You do not have time to think. You just say: let me get to the hospital. Let me find out what is going on.

I drove myself to the ER while having a heart attack.

It is a shocking feeling. One second you are fit and playing tennis with your friend on a beautiful afternoon and the next second you are driving yourself to an emergency room with a piece of paper that says your heart is not working right. There is no transition and no warning and no gradual decline. You are on the tennis court and then you are in the ER. That fast. That sudden. That is what heart disease does. It hides. It waits. And then it announces itself all at once.

I walked into Stamford Hospital and went to the front desk and told them I thought I had had a heart attack. When you say those words, they do not make you wait. They took me back immediately. They drew blood. And then a doctor came in and said the words that divided my life into before and after.

Your troponin level is seven. Something has happened to your heart. We need to keep you overnight.

Troponin is the protein your heart releases when its muscle is damaged. A normal level is near zero. Mine was seven.

I lay in that hospital bed in Stamford, Connecticut. The same town where I had built my life. The same town where my kids went to school and my wife was waiting at home and my tennis racket was still in the car. The same town where I played tennis every week and had beers with my friends and ate low-fat yogurt because my doctor said it was good for my heart.

And I did not understand. How does a professional athlete have a heart attack at 52? How does the fittest guy in the room end up in the ER? How does a man who played at Wimbledon, who never smoked, who exercised every day, who went to every checkup, who did everything the system told him to do. How does that man end up lying in a hospital bed with a troponin of seven and a nurse telling him something has happened to his heart?

Nobody could answer that question. Not that night. Not the next morning. Not during the procedures that followed. Stents went in. A statin prescription came out. Follow-up in three months. No genetic testing. No thyroid investigation. No deep dive into why.

Just: lower the number. Take the pill. See you in three months.

I walked out of that hospital with a bag of drugs and a sentence. You have heart disease. You will be on medication for the rest of your life. Your cholesterol is the problem. We have fixed what we can fix. Manage what we tell you to manage. Do not ask too many questions.

I was 52 years old. And the sport that had defined my entire life since I was six years old in Johannesburg had just tried to kill me.

I did not know it yet. But everything I believed was about to come apart.

CHAPTER 7

THE PILL

I WATCHED THEM PUT THE STENT IN.

I need to tell you what that morning was like. Because unless you have been wheeled into a cath lab on a gurney, you do not know what it feels like to hand your life to a room full of strangers and a screen.

I woke up in the hospital the morning after the ER. They did an ultrasound. Something had happened to my heart. They needed to go in and look. They told me they were taking me to the cath lab.

They wheeled me out of my room and down a hallway and parked me outside the lab. I lay there on my back. On a white sheet. Staring at the ceiling. For about an hour. Because other emergencies came in. Other heart attacks. People who were worse than me. People who needed the lab first.

And I lay there thinking: this is me. This is actually me.

I looked around at the doctors and nurses moving through the hallway. And I realized something that made the whole thing feel like a dream. I was one of the fittest people in the building. Patients, staff, everyone. I was lying on a gurney waiting for heart surgery and I looked healthier than most of the people walking past me on their feet.

People came up to me. Nurses. Technicians. They looked at me and said: wow, you are really fit. It is bizarre that you had a heart event. They kept saying it. Over and over. You do not look like you should be here.

I did not know the word for what I was yet. I would learn it later from Dr. Cywes. TOFI. Thin Outside, Fat Inside. A body that looks healthy while the metabolism is falling apart. I was a textbook case. And nobody in that hospital, including me, knew it.

Then they wheeled me in.

The cath lab is not what you imagine. It is not an operating room with soft lighting and quiet music. It is a lab. Cold. Bright. Technical. They put you on a table. Flat on your back. You cannot move. Above you is a screen. A massive screen. The biggest television you have ever seen, and it is about to show you the inside of your own body.

They made a small cut in my wrist. And they fed a wire through it. A thin metal wire that traveled through my veins and into my heart.

I asked the doctor: am I going to be awake for this?

He said: yes. You will be a little sleepy. But you will see everything.

They gave me something. A mild sedation. Enough to take the edge off. Not enough to put me out. I was conscious. Alert. Lying on a table watching a giant screen showing my own heart pumping in real time.

Every few seconds I would see a burst of dye flood through my veins. Contrast dye. It lit up the arteries so the doctor could see where the blood was flowing and where it was not. Each pulse of dye revealed another branch of the map inside my chest.

The whole thing took maybe 15 or 20 minutes. And then the doctor said the words.

You have a blockage on your LAD artery. The widow maker. We are putting a stent in now.

The widow maker. They call it that because if it closes completely, you die. That is the artery that was narrowing while I ate low-fat yogurt and played tennis and went to my annual checkups and refused statins because I was an athlete and athletes do not have heart problems.

I watched the stent go in. On the screen. A tiny metal cage expanding inside the artery that keeps me alive. I watched it happen to my own heart and I could not process what I was seeing. This was my body. This was the organ that had carried me through Wimbledon and business deals and three children and 52 years of life. And it had been failing without anyone knowing.

My ejection fraction came back at about 50 percent. Normal is around 55. So the damage was not catastrophic. I had gone to the hospital fast. That saved me. Twelve hours between the event on the tennis court and the stent going in. If I had waited another day. If I had told myself it was just heartburn. If I had gone home and gone to bed instead of going to the Tully Center.

I might not be writing this.

They sent me home with a bag of pills. And the first thought was not relief. It was not gratitude that I had survived. It was a question.

Why me?

The second thought was worse.

Can it happen again right now?

That thought never left. Not that day. Not that week. Not for months. It moved into my head like a tenant who refuses to leave. Every minute of every hour. Can I have a heart attack in five minutes? Can I have one in an hour? If I stand up too fast. If I walk too far. If my heart rate goes up. If I breathe too hard.

Is this the moment?

They sent me home with a bag of pills and I started walking.

Not exercise. Not training. Just walking. Around the block. My neighborhood in Stamford. A walk that would take a healthy person ten minutes without thinking about it.

I thought about every step.

I would walk and feel a slight strain and stop. Stand there on the sidewalk. Concentrate on my breathing. Put my hand on my chest. Is my heart okay? Is this normal? Is this what it felt like right before the last one?

I was not living my life. I was monitoring my life. Checking every breath. Testing every heartbeat. Waiting for the next event the way you wait for a second earthquake after the first one. You know it might come. You do not know when. And the not knowing is worse than the event itself.

That is what cardiac fear does to you. It does not just scare you once. It makes you afraid of your own body. The thing that keeps you alive becomes the thing you do not trust. Every chest tightness is a warning. Every moment of breathlessness is a sign. Every heartbeat that feels slightly different is the beginning of the end.

I was 52 years old and I was afraid to walk around my own block.

Then the drug started working. Not the way they intended. The other way.

My cholesterol dropped. That was the goal. The cardiologist wanted 40 and the drug was pushing me there. But cholesterol is not just a number on a lab report. It is a molecule your body uses to build hormones, repair cell membranes, produce vitamin D, and keep your brain functioning. Your liver manufactures it on purpose. Every single day. Because it needs it.

When you crush it to 40, your body does not thank you. Your body breaks.

The memory went first.

80 milligrams of Lipitor. That is what they put me on. And within weeks, something happened to my brain that I did not have the words for at the time. I do now.

It felt like cotton wool had been stuffed inside my head.

My mind, which had always been open and creative, which could think about anything and follow any thread of logic, went dark. Not confused. Not forgetful. Dark. Like a blank screen. I would be walking around my house and I could see what was in front of me. I could process the immediate moment. But beyond that, nothing. No depth. No future thinking. No ability to zoom out and consider anything beyond what I was looking at right now.

It was as if someone had taken a mind that could hold a thousand thoughts and reduced it to one. The one right in front of me. And even that one was hazy.

I would sit in a chair and realize I had no thoughts. Not that I was thinking about nothing. That the mechanism for thinking had stopped. The screen was blank. The filing cabinet was not just empty. The filing cabinet was gone. I could not generate a thought about what happened 10 minutes ago. I could not plan what I was going to do next. I was just there. Sitting. Existing. With cotton wool where my mind used to be.

For a person like me, this was the scariest thing I have ever experienced. More than the heart attack. More than the fear of dying. Because the heart attack was a physical event. It happened and I survived. But the memory loss was an erasure of who I was. I was a creative person. I had built businesses. I could think on my feet. Read a room. Close a deal. Work through complex problems. Play chess with a tennis match. All of that required a mind that could reach into the future and the past simultaneously. And that mind was gone.

My performance at work suffered. I could not hold information. I could not follow a conversation to its conclusion. I would be in a meeting and the first half of the discussion would evaporate before we reached the second half. I would be talking to someone and the word I needed would vanish mid-sentence. Like someone reached into my brain and pulled it out before I could say it.

The fear of losing my intellect caused me enormous anxiety. Not the fear of dying. The fear of losing my mind while still alive. Being trapped inside a body that works with a brain that does not. Walking around with a blank screen in my head for the rest of my life. That was the fear that woke me up at 3 AM worse than any cardiac event.

And I did not connect it to the pill. Because nobody told me to connect it to the pill.

When I mentioned it to my cardiologist, he waved it off. Some people have these effects. Most people are fine. It might be in your head. There might be something else going on.

Something else going on. The man who prescribed a drug that pushes cholesterol to levels the human body was never designed to sustain was telling me the side effects were in my head. The side effects that were in my head were caused by the drug that was destroying my head.

The depression came next.

I need to be specific about this because people use the word depression casually. Bad day at work. Fight with your spouse. A few days of feeling down. That is not what this was.

This was the absence of everything.

The absence of motivation. The absence of joy. The absence of interest in my children, my wife, my work, my friends. The absence of the future. I did not feel sad. I felt nothing. A flat, gray, airless nothing that made every day identical to the one before it and the one after it.

I sat in chairs and did not move. My wife talked to me and the words registered the way background noise registers. Present but meaningless. My kids came home from school and I could not find the energy to ask them a single question about their day.

And underneath all of it, the fear. Still there. Still running. The constant background calculation of whether the next breath would be the last one. Whether the next heartbeat would be the one that stopped.

I was not living. I was dying slowly in a house full of people who loved me and could not reach me.

And then the system offered me something worse.

I had been fighting with my cardiologist about the statins. I could not tolerate them. The memory loss. The aches and pains. The depression. Everything was getting worse, not better. And his answer was not to investigate why. His answer was a new drug.

Repatha.

He told me to try it. A PCSK9 inhibitor. An injectable. Not a pill. A needle. He ordered it and a package arrived at my house in the mail.

I remember opening the package in my bedroom upstairs. I took it out and I looked at it. A prepackaged syringe. A needle. Instructions for injecting yourself.

I almost felt like a junkie.

I sat on the edge of my bed. In my bedroom. In the house where I was supposed to be living my life with my wife and my children. And I took that needle. And I pushed it into my upper thigh. And I injected a foreign substance into my body.

I cannot describe what that moment felt like. I was a professional athlete. I had competed at Wimbledon. I had beaten former world number one players. I had built businesses. I had raised three children. And I was sitting alone in my bedroom pushing a needle into my leg because the medical system had convinced me that my body had let me down. That I was broken. That the only way to survive was to inject a substance into my blood that my body had never asked for and did not need.

I did it twice. Two injections. Two times I sat in that bedroom and pushed a needle into my thigh.

And then I did the research.

The study on Repatha showed that more people had died on the drug than had not. The drug that was supposed to save my life was associated with more deaths. I was injecting myself with a substance that the data said was not working.

But it was not the study that stopped me. It was the needle.

It was the act of sitting in my bedroom and injecting a foreign substance into my body. That was the moment I knew. Not suspected. Not wondered. Knew. Something was profoundly wrong with this system. My body had not let me down. The system had let me down. I was not broken. I was being broken. By pills. By needles. By doctors who answered every question with a new prescription.

I needed to find a way out. I needed to fire my cardiologist. I needed to find another way. Because if the answer to heart disease was sitting in a bedroom alone pushing needles into your leg while your family lived their lives downstairs without you, then the answer was worse than the disease.

My wife Melanie dealt with the worst of it.

She watched me fall. Deeper and deeper. She saw the negativity. The anxiety. The constant focus on my health and my heart. Every conversation was the same. I am not going to make it. I am not going to live. She saw this happen to the man she married. The most positive, optimistic person she knew becoming someone she did not recognize.

And then I said the words.

I told her we needed to get our will in order.

She looked at me and said: Mark, what are you talking about?

I said: Mel, we need to figure out what happens. We need to have everything in place.

She said: You are healthy. You are strong. Why are you saying this? Why are you thinking you are going to die?

I said: Because I am going to die.

And she fought me on it. She would not accept it. She kept saying: you have a family here. Why are you thinking those thoughts? You do not know how long you are going to live. You are strong. You could live a long time. Look at these people who are way worse than you.

Her father, Clive, had had bypass surgery. He was unhealthy. Way more unhealthy than me. And Melanie looked at me and said: you are fit. My father was unhealthy. You are going to last a long time.

But I could not hear it. I was fighting a battle in my mind. She was telling me I was healthy. The fear was telling me I was dying. She was saying look at my father, he was worse. The anxiety was saying it does not matter, you are next. Every piece of logic she offered, the depression swatted away.

She could not fathom what I was saying about the will. About not being alive next week. About planning for my death. She could not process that the man who proposed to her after two and a half weeks, the man who saw what he wanted and went after it, the man who built everything from nothing, was now sitting in their home planning his funeral.

But she did not break. Melanie was the rock.

She fought against me every day. Not with anger. With truth. You are strong. You are doing everything you can. You are going to make it. That is not true. You are not dying. She said it over and over. When I could not say it to myself, she said it for me.

Our relationship was under strain. Not because we stopped loving each other. Because I had become someone she did not marry. The man who had energy for everything had energy for nothing except researching whether he was going to survive the week. Every conversation was heart disease. Every thought was death. I could not talk about the kids. I could not talk about our life. Just the disease. Just the fear. Just the countdown.

It was very hard for her. I know that now. I knew it then, in some distant corner of my mind that could still see outside my own fog. But I could not stop it. The fear and the depression and the memory loss had taken over. And Melanie stood there. Every day. Refusing to let me drown. Telling me the truth when I could not see it myself.

She gave me that support when I needed it most. And I did not know it at the time, but she was keeping me alive as much as any doctor ever would.

Here is what nobody tells you about statins.

Your brain is 25 percent cholesterol by weight. It is the most cholesterol-dense organ in your body. It needs cholesterol to form synaptic connections. To transmit signals. To create the neurotransmitters that regulate your mood, your memory, your ability to think clearly.

When a drug pushes your total cholesterol to 40, your brain does not have the raw material it needs to function. The memory loss is not a coincidence. The depression is not in your head. The cognitive decline is not aging. It is a brain being starved of a molecule it was built to run on.

The Golomb study at UC San Diego documented cognitive side effects in statin users. Memory loss. Confusion. Disorientation. The Wagstaff study in 2003 found cases of amnesia linked to statin use. The evidence was there. My cardiologist either did not know it or did not care.

He wanted the number at 40. He got the number at 40. And he got a patient whose brain was falling apart, whose marriage was under strain, whose children watched their father disappear, and whose will to live had been replaced by a plan to die.

That is what the pill did.

Not to a statistic. Not to a number in a clinical trial. To me. To Melanie. To Sarah. To Rebecca. To David. To everyone who loved me and had to watch me become someone they did not know.

The drug did not save my life. It stole it. And nobody in the system that prescribed it ever acknowledged what was happening.

Until my daughter Sarah walked into the living room and said four words that gave it back.

CHAPTER 8

THE DAUGHTER

I HAD NO WILL TO LIVE.

I need you to understand what that means. I was not sad. Sad is when your team loses or a deal falls through. This was something else entirely. This was a darkness I had never felt in 52 years of living. A heaviness that sat on my chest every morning before I opened my eyes, and a voice in my head that said the same thing every single day.

You are going to die. Not someday. Not eventually. Soon. This week. Maybe today.

I did not know why I had a heart attack. That was the part that destroyed me. If I had been 300 pounds and eating fast food every day, I would have understood. If there had been a history of heart disease in my family, I could have pointed to something and said that is why. But there was nothing. I was the fittest person in every room I walked into. I had played professional tennis on the ATP tour. I played competitive tennis multiple times a week at 52. People standing next to me at the gym were fifty pounds overweight and their hearts were fine.

Yet I was the one on the operating table.

When you do not know why something happened to you, you cannot protect yourself from it happening again. That is the fear. It is not the fear of death. It is the fear of randomness. The feeling that your own body betrayed you for no reason, that it could do it again at any moment, and that there is nothing you can do about it.

So I stopped living.

I was on 80 milligrams of Lipitor. They tried me on Crestor. They tried me on Repatha. Every drug they could find to push my numbers down. My cardiologist wanted my LDL at 40. He wanted to cut it by two thirds from the number my body had always produced.

And I was dying inside. My memory started going. Words I had used my entire life disappeared mid-sentence. I was a creative person who had built businesses and could think on my feet and read a room and close a deal. All of that was gone, replaced by a fog that never lifted. I could not remember what I had for breakfast. I could not follow a conversation. I could not think.

The depression was the worst part. Not sadness. Depression. The kind where you sit in a chair and stare at a wall and do not move. The kind where your wife talks to you and you hear the words but they do not register. The kind where your kids come home from school and you can hear their backpacks dropping on the floor and their voices in the kitchen and you cannot find the energy to ask them about their day.

My father raised me to see every problem as an opportunity. That was how I was built. That was the man who competed at Wimbledon. The man who moved from Johannesburg to California with a tennis racket and a dream and made it work. Positive. Energetic. Present.

That man was gone.

And I did not even know the pills were the reason. Nobody told me. Not my cardiologist, not my primary care doctor, not anyone. The cognitive decline, the depression, the muscle pain, the anxiety. I thought the heart attack had broken something inside me permanently. I thought this was just who I was now. A broken man running out the clock.

Then my daughter Sarah came home.

I was in the living room. I do not remember exactly what day it was or what time. But I remember where I was sitting and I remember the light coming through the window and I remember her face when she walked in.

She sat down across from me. And she looked me in the eyes. And she said:

> *Dad. You are not the same father I have known. You are negative. You are angry. You think you are going to die every second. You are pessimistic. You are not nice to be around. This is not who you are.*

My own daughter. Sarah. The girl I had raised. The girl I had driven to school and helped with homework and taught to never give up. The girl who watched me compete on tennis courts around the world and believed her father could do anything. Sarah was sitting across from me telling me that the man she grew up with had disappeared, and that the person in front of her was someone she did not recognize.

I looked at her.

And something broke open. Not broke down. Broke open. Like a crack in a wall that lets the light through. In that moment I did not feel sad. I felt clarity. The first clarity I had felt since the operating table.

I have to find a way out of here.

That was the thought. Not I should try a different doctor. Not maybe I need therapy. The thought was: there is another way out of this besides these drugs. There has to be. And I am going to find it.

My daughter did not give me medical advice that day. She did not tell me to stop the statin. She did not hand me a study or a book or a doctor's name. She did something harder than any of that.

She told me the truth.

And the truth was that the drugs that were supposed to save my life had taken my life away. In that moment, sitting in my living room, looking at my daughter's face with the afternoon light falling across the floor between us, I made a decision. It was not a medical decision and it was not a scientific decision. It was the simplest decision I had ever made.

If I am going to die, I am going to die as myself.

Not as this ghost. Not as this angry, depressed, hollow version of the man I used to be. If I have a week or a month or a year, I am going to spend it as the father my daughter remembers. The person I was before the pills stole me from my own family. Even if it killed me. I would rather die on my own terms, as the man I was, than live for thirty more years as someone my daughter did not recognize.

That was the fork in the road.

I chose.

My daughter Sarah saved my life that day. Not because she gave me a solution but because she gave me a reason to fight. She held up a mirror and showed me what the system had done to me. And she refused to let me disappear.

She saved my life by telling me the truth.

Everything that happened after that moment. The firing. The research. The doctors. The reversal. The platform. All of it traces back to Sarah sitting across from her father in a living room in Stamford, Connecticut, saying four words that changed everything.

I want my old dad back.

Author's note: This chapter is intentionally short. What happened next belongs to the chapters that follow. This chapter belongs to Sarah. She earned it.

CHAPTER 9

THE FIRING

THE FIRST DRUG WAS LIPITOR. Eighty milligrams. The highest dose they make.

Within weeks I could feel myself disappearing. The memory loss and the depression and the fog that turned every day into the same gray blur. I went back to my cardiologist and told him I could not tolerate it. He did not investigate why. He did not ask what symptoms I was experiencing. He did not consider that the drug might be the problem.

He switched me to Crestor. Forty milligrams. Same thing. Different brand name. Same darkness.

Then Repatha. An injectable. A newer drug, more expensive, same goal. Push the number down. Push it lower. Push it lower than it has ever been in the history of your body and do not ask questions about what happens when you get there.

My cardiologist wanted my LDL at 40.

I need you to sit with that number. Forty. My LDL had always been around 110, the number my liver produced naturally, the number my body chose. He wanted to cut it by two thirds with drugs I could not tolerate, for a reason nobody had explained to me beyond five words: your bad cholesterol is high.

And I was dying inside.

But something else was happening at the same time. Even through the fog, even with a memory that could barely hold a sentence together, something in me was still fighting. I started searching. Late at night, on my phone, on Google, typing with my thumbs the way a drowning man grabs at anything that floats.

> *Natural ways to cure heart disease.*
> *Heart attack causes beyond cholesterol.*
> *Why did I have a heart attack with normal cholesterol.*

I was not a scientist and I was not a doctor. I was a 52-year-old man who had just had a heart attack and could not tolerate the only treatment his cardiologist believed in. I was desperate. And desperate people search harder than anyone.

That is when I found the JUPITER trial.

JUPITER was a massive clinical study. Thousands of patients. Published in a major journal. And what it showed rocked me. It showed that inflammation was a primary driver of heart disease. Not cholesterol. Inflammation. A marker called hs-CRP that my cardiologist had never once ordered. I remember reading that study on my phone in the dark and feeling something I had not felt since before the heart attack.

Hope.

If inflammation was a driver, then maybe cholesterol was not the whole story. If cholesterol was not the whole story, then maybe crushing it to 40 with drugs that were destroying me was not the only path. Maybe there was something else going on, something nobody had looked for, something I could actually fix.

I sent the study to my cardiologist. I emailed him the JUPITER trial, the full study, highlighted the relevant sections, and wrote him a message saying: look, I am seeing things in here that are not about cholesterol. There are other factors. Inflammation. Do I really have to lower my cholesterol to 40?

Then we got on a call. And I will never forget what he said.

His tone changed. He said: Listen, Mark. These are the studies. There is a lot of money behind this. Everyone knows this. Everyone knows that cholesterol is the problem. Who are you? How can you even read these studies? This is what the studies at Pfizer say. Lipitor is proven. It has been proven for 20, 30 years. What are you talking about?

Who are you.

A cardiologist. A man I was trusting with my life. A man I was paying to keep me alive. And his response to a patient bringing him a peer-reviewed clinical trial was: who are you to question this?

Not let me look at that study. Not interesting, let me check your hs-CRP. Not there are actually multiple risk factors and we should investigate further.

Who are you.

He got angry with me. Not concerned. Not curious. Angry. Because I had done something patients are not supposed to do. I had read the science myself. And the science did not say what he had been telling me.

I kept digging and he kept pushing the drugs and I kept asking questions and he kept getting irritated. We were in a fight now. Doctor versus patient. Except the patient had a tennis player's stubbornness and nothing left to lose.

And I thought: if their own study is saying this, what else are they not telling me?

I found the biggest lie of all sitting inside the studies they used to justify the drugs they gave me.

When my cardiologist prescribed Lipitor, and then Crestor, and then Repatha, the argument was always the same. The studies show a 36 percent risk reduction. Take the drug. Reduce your risk by a third. That sounds compelling. That sounds like a drug worth taking. That sounds like the difference between living and dying.

And that is exactly what they wanted it to sound like.

Because the 36 percent is not what you think it is. It is something called relative risk reduction. And relative risk reduction is the single greatest marketing tool the pharmaceutical industry has ever invented.

Let me explain this so a ten year old could understand it, because once you see it, you cannot unsee it.

Imagine a study with two groups of people. In the first group, 3 out of 100 people have a heart attack. In the second group, which takes the drug, 2 out of 100 people have a heart attack. The drug prevented one heart attack out of a hundred people.

One out of a hundred. That is the absolute risk reduction. One percent.

But that is not what they tell you. They take the difference between 3 and 2, which is 1, and they divide it by the original number, which is 3. One divided by three is 33 percent. And so the press release says: this drug reduces your risk of heart attack by 33 percent.

Same data. Different story.

The 33 percent sounds like a miracle. The 1 percent sounds like what it is. A drug that does almost nothing for almost everyone who takes it.

That is what they did with statins. That is what they presented to the FDA. That is what my cardiologist was trained on. That is what he repeated to me when he said take the drug. He was not lying. He believed it. Because the pharmaceutical companies had framed the data so that a one percent benefit looks like a thirty-six percent shield.

When I dug deeper, I found the number that should have been on every prescription bottle in America.

NNT. Number needed to treat. It answers a simple question. How many people need to take this drug for one person to benefit?

For statins in primary prevention, the answer is 200.

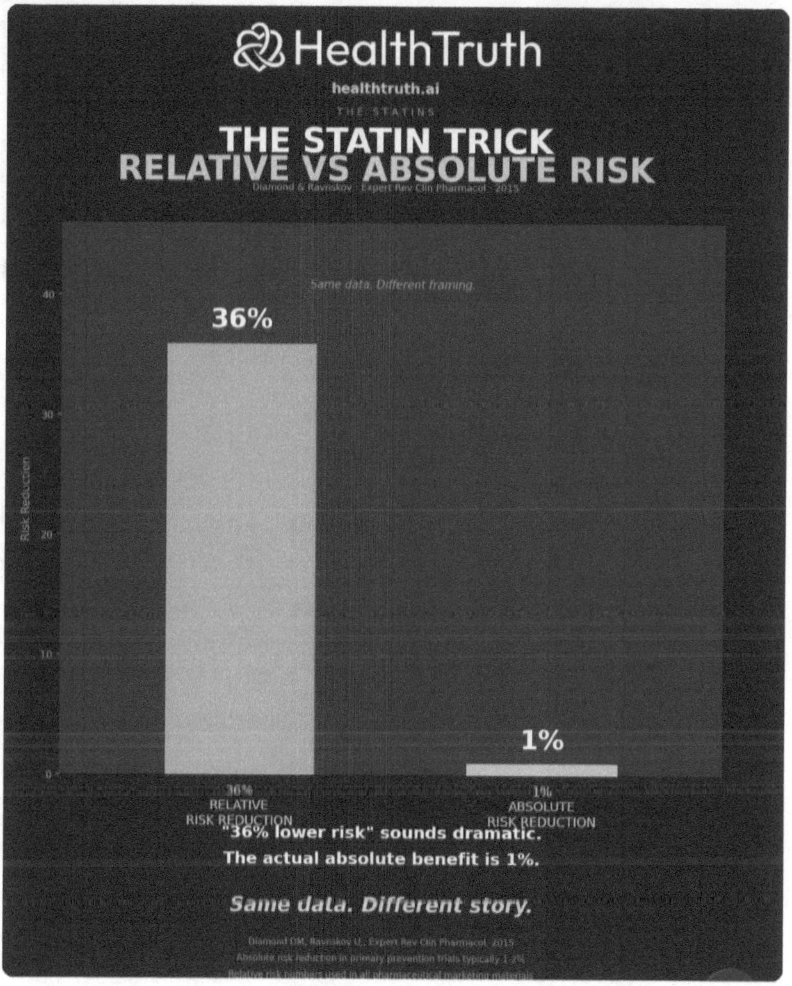

Diamond DM, Ravnskov U. Expert Review of Clinical Pharmacology, 2015. Relative vs absolute risk reduction in statin trials.

Two hundred people take the drug every single day for years. One of them benefits. The other 199 get the side effects, the muscle pain, the memory loss, the depression, the metabolic damage. And they get zero benefit. None. They took the drug for nothing.

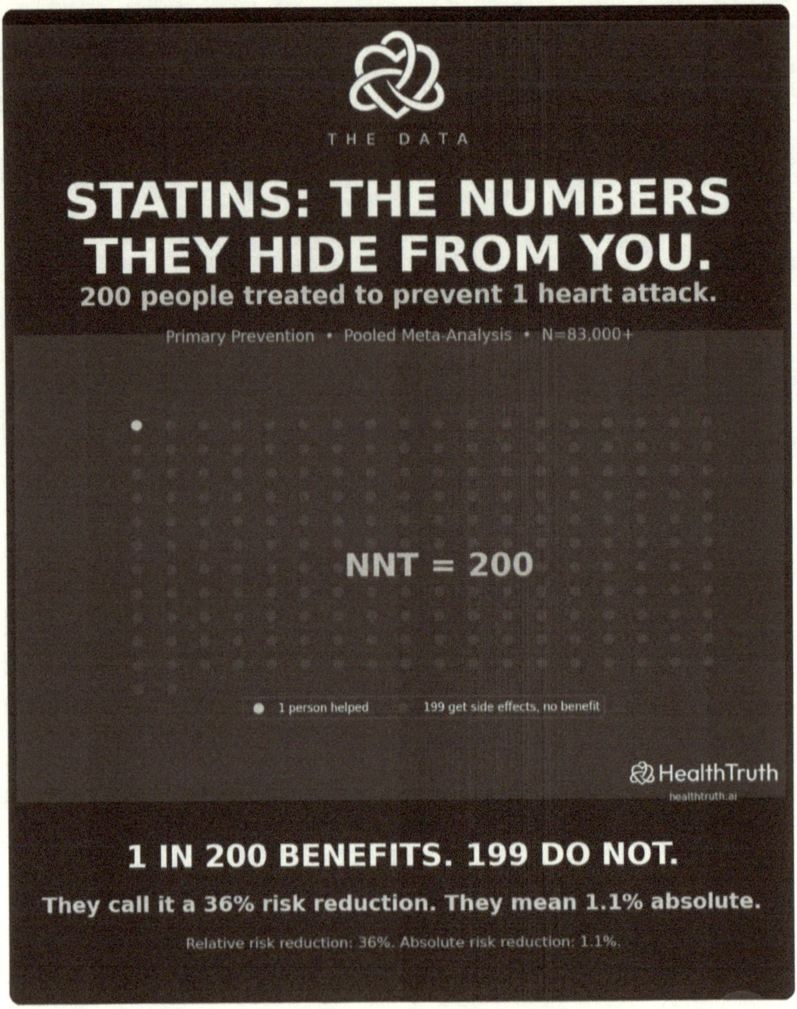

Primary prevention pooled meta-analysis. N>83,000. Number Needed to Treat = 200.

Now stop and think about what that means from a business perspective. Because I have spent 25 years in the insurance industry. I sell products. I know what it takes to bring a product to market, to get it approved by regulators, to convince people to buy it, and to keep them buying it year after year.

If I brought a product to my board that performed like this, one in 200 people benefit and the other 199 get nothing or get worse, that product would be dead on arrival. It would be demolished. Pulled from the shelf. Investigated. My company would face lawsuits. My regulators would shut it down. No insurance product in the history of the industry has ever survived numbers that bad.

But Lipitor did. Crestor did. The statin class did. These became the biggest selling drugs in the history of the pharmaceutical industry. Lipitor alone generated over 125 billion dollars in lifetime revenue. The biggest selling drug in the world. With a one in 200 benefit.

Just sit with that for a moment.

How do you sell a product with almost zero absolute benefit and terrible side effects? Memory loss. Muscle pain. Depression. Diabetes. Cognitive decline. How do you take a product that would be destroyed in any other industry on earth and turn it into the most prescribed drug class in human history?

You have to brainwash an entire system.

You fund the medical schools. You fund the research. You fund the guidelines committees. You fund the continuing education that doctors are required to attend. You train an entire generation of cardiologists to believe that one number is the only number that matters and that your drug is the only answer. You use relative risk reduction to make the data look thirty-six times better than it actually is. You market directly to consumers on television, in magazines, in waiting rooms. You build relationships with insurance companies so the drug is covered and the doctor is penalized for not prescribing it.

That is not medicine. That is the most successful marketing campaign in the history of any industry. And the product it sells has a one in 200 success rate.

I know marketing. I know sales. I know what it takes to move a product. And when I looked at the statin data through the eyes of a businessman instead of a patient, I did not see a medical breakthrough. I saw the greatest fraud in medical history. A product that would not survive a single quarter in any other industry, wrapped in enough institutional support and statistical manipulation to become the standard of care for 92 million Americans.

Then the USPSTF, the United States Preventive Services Task Force, published a systematic review that made it even clearer. Out of 100 people who take statins for five years, 97.8 get nothing. No benefit at all. 1.2 are helped. And 1 gets diabetes. From the drug. The drug that was supposed to protect them gave almost as many people a new disease as it helped.

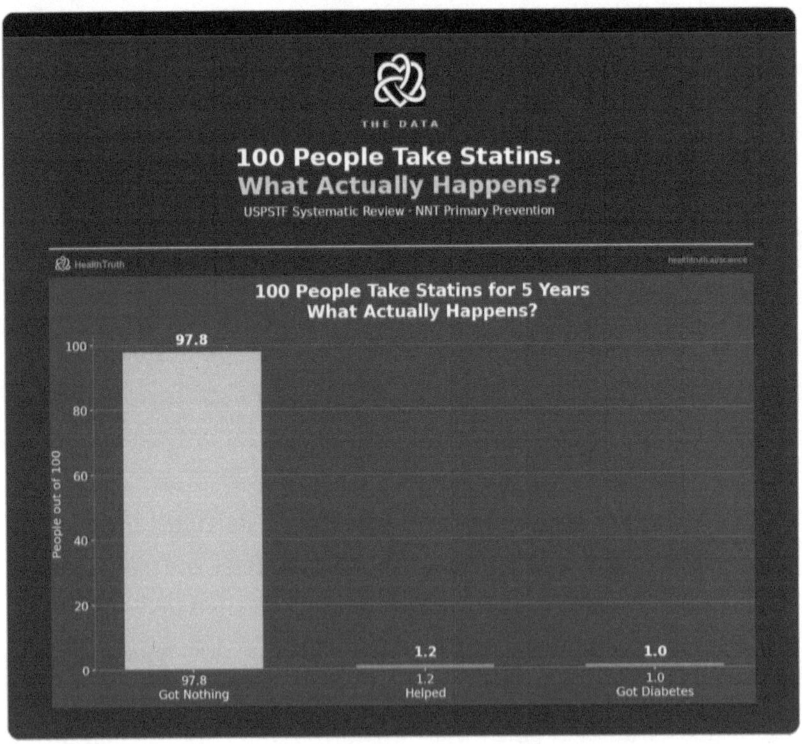

USPSTF Systematic Review. Statin use for primary prevention of cardiovascular disease in adults.

And here is the part that should make your blood boil. It was not just statins.

I looked at the Repatha study. The PCSK9 inhibitor. The needle I pushed into my thigh in my bedroom while my family lived their lives downstairs. The same trick. Relative risk reduction in the headlines. Absolute risk reduction buried in the data. The benefit was marginal. The marketing was spectacular.

But the Repatha data was worse than marginal. The FOURIER trial studied 27,564 patients. When the BMJ Open readjudicated the data in 2022, the results were staggering. 113 cardiac deaths on Repatha. 88 on placebo. Twenty-eight percent more people died on the drug than on nothing. The drug my cardiologist called the future. The needle I pushed into my thigh because the system told me it was the next generation of heart protection. More people died on it.

My cardiologist called this drug the future. The data called it a failure.

This is how the pharmaceutical industry works. The data is so bad that they have to put lipstick on it. They have to use relative risk reduction because if they reported the absolute numbers, no doctor would prescribe the drug and no patient would take it. They frame the data to get FDA approval. Then they train the doctors on the framing. Then the doctors repeat the framing to the patients. And the patients swallow the pills.

I was one of those patients. Swallowing pills that had a one percent absolute benefit while my cardiologist told me they reduced my risk by a third.

But the lie does not stop at the doctor's office. It goes deeper.

I learned something that most patients never find out. When I go to see my doctor and my cholesterol is 120, the system expects my doctor to prescribe a statin. Not suggest. Not consider. Prescribe. If my doctor does not flag my cholesterol and write that prescription, the insurance company flags the doctor. The doctor gets dinged on their performance report. They are marked as non-compliant with the guidelines.

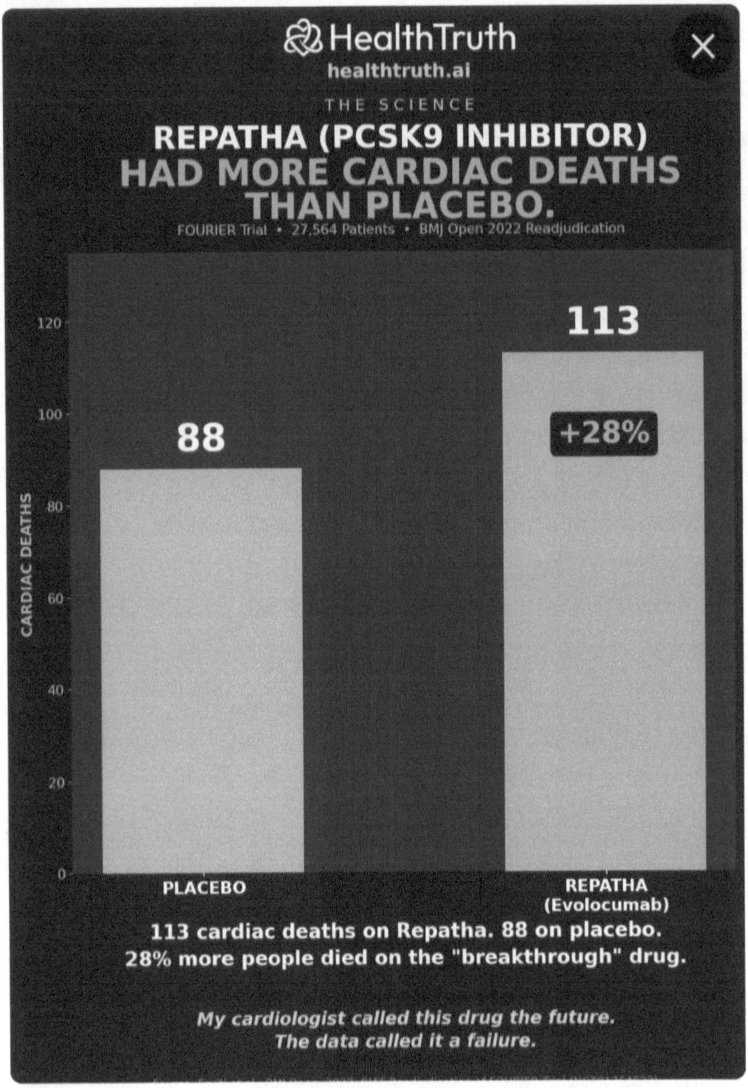

Erviti J et al., BMJ Open, 2022. Readjudication of cardiac mortality data from the FOURIER trial. N=27,564.

Think about what that means. The insurance companies are connected to the drug companies. The drug companies train the doctors. The guidelines are built on relative risk reduction data that makes a one percent benefit look like a thirty-six percent miracle. And if a doctor looks at the absolute data and decides that their patient does not need the drug, the system punishes them.

The doctor is not free to practice medicine. The doctor is free to practice the guidelines. And the guidelines were written by people with financial ties to the companies that make the drugs.

This is not health care. This is sick care. A system designed to prescribe a drug with almost no absolute benefit, funded by companies that profit from the prescription, enforced by insurance companies that penalize doctors who do not comply, and marketed with a statistical trick that makes the whole thing sound like science.

And if 92 million Americans are taking this drug, and heart disease is still the number one killer on the planet, then the biggest question is not whether statins work.

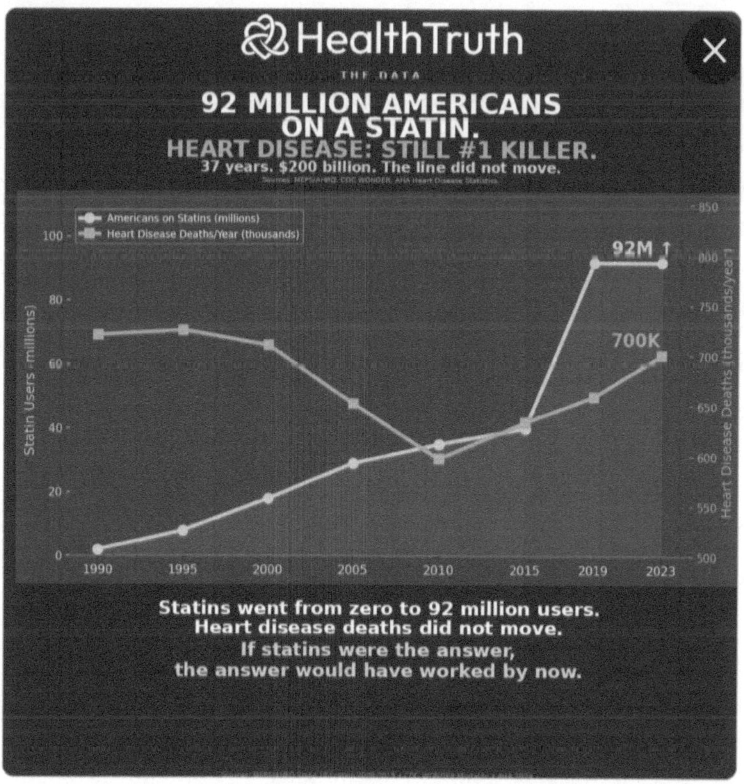

Sources: MEPS/AHRQ Statin Utilization 2008–2019. CDC WONDER Mortality Data. AHA Heart Disease Statistics, 2024.

The biggest question is why nobody is asking why they do not.

That was the lie. And once I saw it, I could not unsee it. Every study. Every drug. Every headline that said reduces risk by 30 percent. I knew what they were doing. I knew the real number. And I knew that the system that had given me these drugs, that had crushed my cholesterol to 40, that had stolen my memory and my personality and my will to live, had done it based on a statistical trick that a ten year old could see through if anyone bothered to show them the math.

Nobody showed them the math. Until now.

And then the logic hit me. If statins were curing heart disease, why is heart disease still the number one killer on the planet?

Then I did something I did not tell him about.

I went upstairs to my bathroom, took the pill bottles out of the cabinet, Lipitor, Crestor, all of them, and opened them over the toilet. I watched the pills swirl and disappear into the water, carrying with them every morning I had reached into that cabinet and put a toxin into my body because a doctor told me to.

I pulled the chain.

That was my signal. I was done. Done with these poison pills. Every time I looked at that pill box I knew they were killing me. They were the drugs that stole my memory. I was reliant on a synthetic substance and I did not believe, deep down, that it was going to heal me. We were not born statin deficient. Why was I taking this drug?

I stood in my bathroom and I felt something I had not felt in months.

Freedom.

The dependency was gone. The daily ritual of swallowing a pill that made me feel like hell was over. No more reaching into the medicine cabinet every morning and putting a toxin into my body. If you look at how statins were discovered, it was a mycotoxin, a mold found in Asia. That is what I had been putting into my body every day. A toxin. And now it was gone. Flushed. Down the toilet. Out of my life.

I was on my own. No drug, no cardiologist supporting me, no safety net. Just me and the research and the deep belief that the natural way was the way to heal. I was going to solve this. Not with a synthetic drug. With food and science and the fuel my body was designed to run on.

It was the happiest day I had had since the heart attack.

I was set free.

And something else happened that I did not expect. When the drug left my body, my father came back. Not him. His gift. The optimism, the belief that there is always some water in the glass. The statins had taken that from me. They had turned the most positive person in the room into someone my wife and daughter did not recognize. That was not me. That was the drug. And when I flushed it, I got my father's son back.

A few weeks later, I had to do my routine bloodwork. I went to the lab and they drew the vials and the results went to my cardiologist.

My cholesterol had gone back up. Back to around 100. He knew immediately.

The phone rang. And I will never forget his voice.

Mark. You are not taking the drug.

It was not a question. He could see it in the numbers. The number he had spent months trying to crush to 40 had climbed back to where my body wanted it. The evidence was in the blood draw.

I told him the truth. I told him I could not do it anymore.

And he said the words that I carry with me to this day.

You could die tomorrow. You could die on Monday of a heart attack. And you better take that drug.

You could die on Monday.

A doctor. My doctor. The man who was supposed to be my partner in staying alive. And his final argument was not science and it was not data and it was not a study or a scan or a test result. It was fear. Take the drug or die.

That was the moment. Not the heart attack. Not the ER. Not the stents. This phone call. This sentence. This doctor choosing fear over curiosity. Choosing a number over a patient. Choosing the guideline over the human being on the other end of the line.

I fired him.

Not in some dramatic scene. Not with a speech. I just never went back. I hung up the phone and I knew. I was done with the system. Done with the drugs. Done with a model of medicine that could not answer a single question about why I had a heart attack but was absolutely certain that crushing one number with a pill I could not tolerate was the only thing standing between me and death.

I was terrified. I want to be honest about that. I was not brave and I was not confident. I was a 52-year-old man with a recent heart attack, no cardiologist, no medical team, and no plan. I had just been told by a credentialed physician that I could die on Monday.

And I had chosen to walk away.

But I had also seen something he did not want me to see. I had seen the JUPITER trial. I had seen that inflammation mattered. I had seen that the cholesterol story had cracks in it. Small cracks. But cracks. And cracks are where the light gets in.

My daughter had given me the reason to fight. The JUPITER trial had given me the first piece of evidence that the fight was worth having. And my cardiologist, by choosing fear and anger over science and curiosity, had shown me that the system I was trusting with my life was not interested in the truth.

It was interested in the number.

I unplugged. Not because I was sure I would survive. Not because I had a better plan. Because the plan they had was killing me. And dying as myself was better than surviving as a ghost.

I had no doctor. No roadmap. No team. I had a phone and a Google search bar and the stubbornness of a man who once played at Wimbledon.

It would have to be enough.

PART THREE

THE UNPLUG

THE SIX-YEAR INVESTIGATION.
THE DOCTORS WHO RISKED EVERYTHING.
THE SCIENCE THEY BURIED.
THE REVERSAL THEY SAID WAS IMPOSSIBLE.

CHAPTER 10

THE DARK HOLE

I DID NOT THINK I WAS GOING TO MAKE IT PAST A WEEK.

That is not a metaphor and it is not the kind of thing people say to describe a difficult time. I mean that I woke up every morning genuinely believing that this could be my last day alive. I had fired my cardiologist, I had stopped my medication, and the last words a medical professional had said to me were: you could die on Monday.

It was dark. The darkest place I have ever been. Darker than the heart attack itself, because at least during the heart attack someone was in charge. Doctors were moving, machines were beeping, stents were going in. Someone had a plan.

Now nobody had a plan. I had no doctor, no team, no protocol. Just a phone and a search bar and a fear that sat on my chest heavier than any cardiac event.

I needed one thing. The only thing that could keep me alive long enough to figure this out.

I needed hope.

Hope, for me, was not a motivational quote or a book title or a podcast or a friend telling me everything was going to be okay. Hope was proof. Proof that people like me had survived. That someone with my markers, my genetics, my history had made it through and was still alive years later. Not just surviving. Living.

Because if they existed, then I could exist.

So I went looking for them. I started on Facebook, joining every heart disease group I could find, and there were dozens of them, hundreds. Groups for heart attack survivors, for people with high Lp(a), for people with APOE e4, for people questioning statins, for people who had fired their cardiologists and were trying to figure out what to do next.

I was not there to post. I was there to read.

I would sit at my dining room table after my family went to bed. Melanie and the kids upstairs. The house quiet except for the hum of the refrigerator and the occasional creak of the floorboards above me. And I would open my laptop and disappear.

I found Dr. William Davis's forum first. He was a cardiologist who had written about the dangers of wheat and the limitations of the cholesterol hypothesis. His forum had been running since about 2004. Sixteen years of data. Sixteen years of people posting their blood work, their genetics, their progress, their setbacks. Thousands of threads and thousands of lives documented in real time across nearly two decades.

I had never seen anything like it. This was not a study published in a journal. This was real people with real names and real numbers, tracked over years, and all of it was just sitting there, open, waiting for someone like me to find it.

I started searching for people with my genetics. APOE e3/e4. High Lp(a). A cardiac event. And I would follow their thread, not for a few posts but for years, starting at their first post and scrolling forward through every update, every lab result, every question they asked, every answer they received. For hours.

There was a man named Carl.

Carl had the same genetics as me. He had started posting on the forum around 2004. I picked up his thread and I followed him year by year, post by post. His blood work, his supplements, his diet changes, his setbacks, his progress. I followed him through sixteen years of his life on that forum.

And then I found him in 2021. Still posting. Still alive.

I was sitting at my dining room table at 2 AM and I almost cried. Here was a man with my genetics, APOE e3/e4, high Lp(a), the same loaded gun, and he had been carrying it for sixteen years and he was still here. Still fighting. Still living.

That was the first time I thought: I can survive this.

Then I found Pat.

Pat's story was the one that gave me the most hope of anyone on the forums. He had been working in corporate, went in for a routine physical at one of the top hospitals, and they came back with news that would have destroyed most people. His main artery was calcified, severely, and they told him he had maybe a year, maybe less. His heart was a ticking bomb and the medical system had no answer other than surgery and drugs.

But Pat was an engineer. And engineers solve problems.

He spent the next year doing what no doctor expected him to do. He figured out how the body worked, went deep into the science of arterial calcification, and discovered something that the cardiology establishment was not focused on. Vitamin K2. A vitamin that directs calcium into your bones and teeth and away from your arteries. A vitamin that most people have never heard of and that was the missing piece.

This was the early 2000s and nobody was talking about K2. Pat was ahead of the science by a decade. He started supplementing and then he did something remarkable. He tracked his calcium with CT scans, not yearly but every three to four months, scan after scan after scan, watching the number.

And over time, the calcium in his artery went down. He reduced it. Then he eliminated it.

The medical community says you cannot reverse coronary calcium.

Pat did it.

An engineer with no medical degree figured out what cardiologists could not. And he documented every step on William Davis's forum.

Pat wrote a manifesto and laid out his entire philosophy of heart disease, and he called it the 12-Headed Dragon. Because heart disease is not one thing. It is not just cholesterol. It is a dragon with twelve heads. Thyroid, insulin resistance, inflammation, Lp(a), vitamin D, K2 deficiency, homocysteine, and more. You cannot kill the dragon by cutting off one head. The system tries to kill one head with a statin. The other eleven keep breathing fire.

That manifesto changed how I understood my own disease. It was not cholesterol. It was everything.

Pat built a vitamin business called Concentrated K and turned his research into a product. He was not just a survivor. He was a builder. Like me. An engineer who solved his own problem and then built something to help others solve theirs.

And then Pat did something for me personally that I will never forget.

We connected and we chatted and he looked at my situation and he said: Mark, you need thyroid. Your thyroid is not right. Thyroid is a big driver for you. You need Armour Thyroid.

Armour Thyroid is ground-up thyroid gland, a natural supplement, not a synthetic drug. The kind of treatment that functional medicine doctors prescribe but mainstream cardiologists never mention.

Pat sent me some of his own supply. Because I had to order it and it was going to take time and he did not want me to wait. A stranger on a forum. A man in his sixties who had been told he was going to die twenty years earlier, sending me his own thyroid supplement because he knew I needed it now.

I took it and it changed how I felt almost immediately. My energy shifted. My body temperature regulated. The fog continued to lift. Thyroid had been flagged four times on my blood panels.

Four times. And no doctor had ever addressed it. Pat, an engineer I found on a forum at 2 AM, addressed it with a package in the mail.

And then I found Fred.

I was searching a Facebook group late one night, scrolling through posts the way I had been scrolling for weeks, looking for proof that people like me survived. And there was Fred. Eighty years old. Still active. Still posting. Still alive.

His story was the one that made me believe the body can heal itself.

Fred had gone to his doctor about 30 years earlier, around age 50, with angina. Chest pain. The kind that stops you in your tracks and makes you think this is it. His doctor told him what every doctor tells you. You need surgery. You need drugs. You need to get into the system.

Fred walked out.

He did not take the drugs. He did not go in for the surgery. He went home and he started exercising. In his bedroom. In his bathroom. Jump rope. Bodyweight exercises. Nothing fancy. No gym membership. No trainer. A man with chest pain, in his house, jumping rope.

And the angina went away.

That is the part that sounds impossible until you understand what was happening. Fred changed his food. He cut out the processed garbage. He ate real food. He moved his body. And over time, his body did what bodies are designed to do when you give them the right fuel and the right movement. It healed.

Thirty years later, I found him in a Facebook group running his own protocol page, sharing what he had learned with strangers who were as scared as I was. No angina. No surgery. No drugs. Eighty years old and living proof that the system's prognosis is not your destiny.

I reached out to him. I messaged him the same way I had messaged Carl and Pat. And he called me back. And talking to Fred was one of the most amazing conversations I have ever had. Here was a man who had stared at the same fear I was staring at, who had been told by a doctor that he needed to get into the system or die, who had chosen a different path, and who was still here 30 years later to tell me about it.

Carl gave me proof that my genetics were survivable. Pat gave me the science and the protocol. Fred gave me something else. Fred gave me proof that the body wants to heal. That if you remove the poison and give it the right fuel, it will do the work. That the system is not the only path. That sometimes the bravest thing a patient can do is trust their own body more than they trust the prescription.

Pat is still alive. He is in his seventies. It has been almost twenty-five years since they told him his artery was calcified and he had a year to live. Twenty-five years. Still here. Still helping people. Still proving that the system's prognosis is not your destiny.

That is who saved me. Not the medical system. Not the cardiologist. Not the hospital. Carl. Pat. Fred. Strangers on forums who understood what I was going through because they had been through it themselves.

But it was not just the forums. It was the books. And one Google search.

Once the Lipitor was gone and my memory started coming back, it was amazing how quickly my mind returned. The cotton wool dissolved and the blank screen came back to life. And the first thing I did with my mind was read.

I read everything. I could not stop. Dr. Stephen Sinatra's books, Dr. Aseem Malhotra's A Statin-Free Life, Philip Ovadia's Stay Off My Operating Table, Dr. William Davis's work. Every book led me to another book and every book opened up more ideas, more search terms, more threads to pull.

And every book confirmed what the JUPITER trial had shown me, the study I had found and sent to my cardiologist before he asked me who I was to question the science. It was not just cholesterol. It was never just cholesterol. The books opened up more search terms, more threads to pull, more evidence that the thing the system was treating was not the thing that was killing people.

If statins were curing heart disease, why is heart disease still the number one killer on the planet? Billions of dollars spent. Hundreds of millions of prescriptions written. Decades of the entire medical system focused on lowering cholesterol. And heart disease is still number one. Nothing added up.

There was one more doctor who changed my path. And I managed to speak to him before he died.

Dr. Stephen Sinatra was a cardiologist who wrote three books that I read cover to cover. He was one of the first mainstream cardiologists to say publicly that cholesterol was not the driver, that inflammation and metabolic dysfunction and nutritional deficiencies were the real causes. He developed the Sinatra Protocol: CoQ10, L-carnitine, D-ribose, magnesium. He was treating heart disease with nutrition, not statins. And his patients were getting better.

I found his phone number. I called him. And he took my call.

I was on Greenwich Avenue in Connecticut. Melanie was in the car with me, the engine running, the windows up. And I was speaking to the man whose books had given me a framework for understanding what had happened to my body. I said: Doctor, I have high Lp(a). What do I need to do? Do you think I will be okay?

And he said: Mark, you will be okay. Manage your inflammation. Take CoQ10. Take lumbrokinase for the clotting. You will be fine.

I sat in the car with Melanie and I felt the most enormous sigh of relief. A cardiologist. A real cardiologist. A man who had spent decades treating heart disease. Telling me I was going to be okay. Not by prescribing a statin. By telling me to manage inflammation and take supplements.

That phone call happened before Stephen Sinatra passed away. I am grateful I got to speak to him and I am grateful he took the call from a stranger. CoQ10 is in my supplement stack to this day because of that conversation on Greenwich Avenue.

My family was sleeping upstairs. And I was sitting at the dining room table at 3 AM, sometimes 4 AM, reading the words of people who had survived what I was going through. And for the first time since the heart attack, I had something I had not had in months.

A plan.

Not a doctor's plan. Not a prescription. Not a protocol handed to me in a ten-minute appointment. My own plan. Built from the evidence of people who had actually made it through. Carl was alive. Pat had reversed his calcium. Fred was in his eighties and still running a forum. These people had done it. Without drugs. Without the system.

And I was going to do it too.

I started reaching out to these people. Not just reading their posts but contacting them, sending messages, texting, emailing, introducing myself as a heart attack survivor who was trying to understand what they had figured out.

And they responded. Almost all of them. Because they remembered what it felt like to be where I was. Terrified. Alone. Searching at 2 AM for proof that life continues after the diagnosis.

They told me what they ate and what they stopped eating and what tests they demanded and what doctors they trusted and what worked and what did not. They were not scientists. They were not doctors. They were patients. Survivors. People who had unplugged from the system and built their own protocols through trial and error and stubbornness.

They were my people.

And through those conversations, something started to form. Not a business plan and not a product idea. A question.

Why is this so hard? Why does a 52-year-old heart attack survivor have to spend five hours a night on Facebook forums tracking strangers to find out if he is going to live? Why is there no place where people with the same genetics, the same markers, the same conditions can find each other and find hope? Why does the medical system hand you a prescription and send you home with no network, no community, no connection to the people who have already been through what you are about to go through?

Why does hope have to be this hard to find?

That question is the genesis of HealthTruth | Neo. Not the technology, not the AI, not the biomarker database or the functional ranges or the root cause framework. Those came later. The thing that started it all was a man sitting alone at his kitchen table at 3 AM, scrolling through a Facebook group, looking for proof that he was going to survive, and thinking: nobody should have to do this alone.

The people I found on those forums saved my life. Carl and Pat and Fred and the strangers on William Davis's forum and the people in the APOE groups and the Lp(a) groups and the statin-questioning groups. They did not know they were saving my life. They were just sharing their stories and posting their numbers and showing up.

But it became more than reading. It became a tribe. I started doing live group calls with them, texting, sharing my labs, listening to theirs. People who were twenty years into heart disease saying: look, Mark, this is how I am eating. I am managing it. I feel great. And just having that community, that close camaraderie, those conversations with people who understood what it felt like to be told you could die on Monday and choose to fight anyway.

It is hard to talk to someone about heart disease when they have never had it. They listen and they nod and they say the right things. But they do not know. They do not know what it feels like to check your pulse at 3 AM because you are not sure your heart is still beating. They do not know the weight of every breath when you believe each one could be your last.

These people knew. They had been there. They were a special club that nobody wants to join, but once you are in it, the bond is unlike anything else. When you have had a heart attack, you are a member of a tribe. And that tribe saved me.

Not just the science. Not just the books. Not just the doctors. The people. Other patients. Other survivors. Humans who had walked through the same fire and come out the other side and were willing to turn around and pull the next person through.

And something else was happening to me as I healed. Something I did not expect.

I was getting angry.

Not the depression anger and not the fear anger. A different kind. The kind that comes from injustice. The kind I used to feel on the tennis court when the calls went against me and I was down two sets and my back was against the wall.

I started to see it clearly. There are mothers out there and fathers and sisters and daughters taking these drugs, getting their cholesterol down to 30, still eating the bagels, still drinking the orange juice, thinking they are safe, thinking the pill is protecting them. And they are dying of heart disease with low cholesterol because nobody told them about the other eleven causes. Nobody tested their insulin or checked their thyroid or looked at their genetics. The system told them one number mattered and they believed it. The same way I believed it.

And that felt like an injustice. Not a medical debate. An injustice. People are being harmed by a system that is supposed to help them. Families are losing people who could have been saved with a $300 blood panel and a conversation about food.

And I made a decision. The same decision I had made a thousand times on a tennis court when I was down and the crowd had counted me out and my opponent thought the match was over.

I am going to fight the system.

Quietly. Patiently. The way the underdog always fights. Build something, build it right, build it to last, and give every person out there who is taking a pill and thinking they are safe the information that could actually save their life.

The anger was fuel. The same fuel that had carried me from middle of the pack at thirteen to Wimbledon. The same fuel that had carried me from the operating table to the research. Now it was carrying me from patient to advocate. From survivor to builder.

I wanted to build that for everyone. A place where anyone who has just been diagnosed, anyone who has just been scared, anyone who has just been handed a bag of pills and told this is their life now, can find hope without spending five hours a night on forums. Where the network of survivors and the science and the doctors and the data are all in one place. Where the first thing you feel when you land there is not fear.

It is hope.

That is who we are. I tried to save my life. I found hope through people who had survived before me. And through those people, I decided to build a global health platform so that nobody else has to search for hope in the dark.

CHAPTER 11

THE DOCTORS WHO RISKED EVERYTHING

I DID NOT FIND THESE DOCTORS BY ACCIDENT.

When you are drowning and you finally break the surface, you do not find land by luck. You find it because you are swimming harder than you have ever swum in your life and you are looking in every direction at once. That is what I was doing at 2 AM on my phone, at 6 AM with a book I could barely read because my memory was still coming back from the statins, on forums where strangers were sharing their blood panels and their stories and their rage.

I was looking for someone. Anyone. Who was telling the truth.

The first truth I found was in a book.

Nina Teicholz wrote a book called The Big Fat Surprise. It was a New York Times bestseller, and it changed my life.

I read that book and I was shocked. Not surprised. Shocked. The kind of shock where you put the book down and stare at the wall and your entire understanding of food rearranges itself in front of you. The book laid out how the foods we have been eating for millions of years on this earth, meat, butter, eggs, animal fat, the foods that sustained every generation of humans that ever lived, had been made into villains. Manufactured into killers. Through manipulated studies and cherry-picked data and Ancel Keys and the Seven Countries Study and the deliberate suppression of evidence that contradicted the low-fat hypothesis.

Millions of years. Humans have been eating these foods for millions of years. And in the space of a few decades, the food industry and the medical establishment convinced the entire world that they were poison. That is not a mistake. That is a manipulation. And Nina Teicholz documented it with the precision of an investigative journalist and the courage of someone who knew the industry would come after her.

They did come after her. The dietary establishment, the food tribes, big food, big pharma. They attacked her credibility and questioned her motives. She is still fighting today. Still publishing. Still telling the truth.

And here is what that book did to me personally.

I went to a steakhouse and I ordered a steak with butter on it. And for the first time in my adult life, I felt no guilt.

None.

I sat there with a beautiful piece of beef in front of me, butter melting on top, and I thought: this food is healing me. Not killing me. Healing me. And I felt the most amazing satisfaction. Not just the taste but the freedom, the release of decades of guilt that the guidelines had put on my shoulders. I was eating a steak with butter and it was good for me. And I knew it because I had read the science.

I had eggs the next morning. With the yolks. And I thought the same thing. This food is healing me.

And here is what I realized as I started eating this way. I was not hungry. That was the surprise. After years of eating rice cakes and bread and drinking grapefruit juice and orange juice and low-fat everything, I was always hungry, always reaching for the next snack, always craving something an hour after a meal. The sugar and the carbohydrates were keeping me on a treadmill of hunger.

A big steak with butter and eggs. There is no way you are eating much after that. I was satiated. Completely. For the first time in my adult life, I finished a meal and did not think about food for hours. The taste of the meat was better and the eggs were better and everything tasted better because my body was getting what it actually needed.

I felt an enormous sense of performance. Not just physical but mental. The fog was lifting and the cotton wool was clearing. I was not on the statin anymore and I was eating the food my body was designed to eat and the combination was bringing me back.

And I kept thinking: why is this not available everywhere? Why are people going to steakhouses and feeling guilty about eating meat? Why is a 55-year-old man at a restaurant afraid to order a steak because his doctor told him saturated fat would kill him? This is what the guidelines have done. They have made people afraid of the food that heals them and replaced it with orange juice and rice cakes and margarine and bread that is slowly making them sick.

I was not addicted to sugar. I did not crave the old foods. Once I started eating steak and eggs, the cravings disappeared because my body was finally getting the fuel it was designed to run on. You do not crave gasoline when the engine is full. You only crave when you are starving.

And I had been starving on a full stomach for thirty years.

Nina Teicholz gave me that. Her book gave me permission to eat the food that would save my life. She is not a co-founder of HealthTruth | Neo. But she is one of the warriors who started this movement. And I owe her a debt I can never repay.

The first doctor I found was Philip Ovadia.

When you fire your cardiologist, the next best thing you can find is a heart surgeon who agrees that the system is broken. There are not many of them. Heart surgeons who question the cholesterol hypothesis, who talk about insulin resistance and metabolic health and root cause medicine. Philip Ovadia is one of the few.

I found him online. He was on Facebook. I did something that most people would not do. I just messaged him on Facebook Messenger. I wrote something like: Dr. Ovadia, my name is Mark Kaplan. I was a former tennis professional. I had a heart event. I need some help.

And he responded back.

The joy I felt when I saw his reply is something I cannot fully describe. A heart surgeon. A real, credible, practicing heart surgeon had responded to a stranger's message on Facebook. I was sitting there looking at my phone and I thought: here is someone who is going to be my partner in healing me.

I am not alone anymore.

I got his email and we exchanged messages and I texted him and then we got on a call. That first call changed everything. Philip listened. He heard my story, the heart attack, the athlete, the statins, the memory loss, the Repatha injections, the firing, all of it. And then he went through my labs.

And here is what I noticed. He was not looking at my LDL.

That was the biggest relief I had felt since the heart attack. He was never going to focus on LDL. My LDL was 110 and it was not even high and every other doctor had been fixated on it. Philip did not care about 110. He cared about what was underneath it.

He went straight to the root cause. My thyroid, my insulin resistance, my inflammation markers. The data that my cardiologist had either disregarded or never tested in the first place. He started to make sense of all the numbers that had been sitting in my labs for years, ignored, while every doctor stared at the one number that did not matter.

Here is someone who is honest. Someone who knows the science. Someone who is focusing on the areas that I had started to discover through my own research at 2 AM on the forums. He was confirming everything I had been piecing together alone, and he was doing it with the authority of a man who had spent over twenty years standing over patients whose hearts had been destroyed by the same metabolic dysfunction he was now finding in my blood.

He had me do more tests, the tests my cardiologist never ordered. I submitted them and we had more calls. And for the first time since the heart attack, I had a path. Not a guess, not a forum thread, not a Google search at 3 AM. A path. Built by a heart surgeon who had held failing hearts in his hands and asked the question that changed his career: why am I operating on these people? What happened upstream that brought them to my table?

Philip wrote a book called Stay Off My Operating Table, and the cover has meats and eggs and fish on it. A heart surgeon telling you to eat the foods that every other doctor says will kill you. When I saw that cover, I thought: there is something happening here. Something is changing. And I want to be part of it.

His book confirmed everything Nina's book had started. Meat, eggs, fish, real food. The food that heals. Coming from a cardiac surgeon who had spent two decades repairing the damage caused by not eating those foods.

Having Philip Ovadia on my team was the most amazing feeling. Not because he told me everything was fine but because he had my back. He was working with me and not against me. He was not trying to sell me a drug. He was trying to find the truth. And he became the genesis of what I would build. HealthTruth | Neo. A platform filled with doctors like Philip. Doctors who look deeper. Doctors who ask why.

The next book I picked up was by Aseem Malhotra. A Statin-Free Life.

I was researching the damage that statins can do. I was looking for evidence that not taking the drug was okay, that I was not committing suicide by stopping my medication. And I found Aseem's book. Reading it was like finding oxygen. Here was a credentialed cardiologist. Not a blogger, not an influencer. A cardiologist trained in the UK medical system who had written an entire book laying out the case that statins are massively overprescribed, that the relative risk reductions marketed to patients are misleading, and that lifestyle intervention outperforms drug intervention for cardiovascular prevention.

He gave me hope that not taking the drug was actually okay. That there were more people out there who had stopped and were doing fine. That the fear my cardiologist had planted in me was not the whole truth.

The British medical establishment came after him for it. They did not challenge his data. They challenged his credibility, his motives, his standing. Because in a system where the pharmaceutical industry funds 70 percent of continuing medical education for doctors, a cardiologist who questions statins is not seen as a scientist. He is seen as a threat.

Aseem Malhotra kept going. He is still going. He is a giant. And I am standing on his shoulders.

Robert Cywes found me through his video content. He is a metabolic surgeon with a PhD, incredibly smart and incredibly detailed, and he said something to me that stopped me cold.

He called me a TOFI. Thin Outside, Fat Inside.

I was not hugely overweight when I had my heart attack. I looked fine. Everyone told me I was in great shape. But Robert Cywes explained that you can be thin on the outside and metabolically destroyed on the inside. Visceral fat, fatty liver, insulin resistance, all hidden beneath a body that looks healthy.

I was drinking orange juice and grapefruit juice every morning thinking it was healthy, and I was becoming insulin resistant from the fructose in those drinks alone. The fruit juice that every nutritionist recommends was quietly destroying my metabolism.

Robert Cywes calls sugar and refined carbohydrates what they are. An addiction. Same neural pathways as alcohol, same dopamine and opioid responses, same denial, same relapse patterns. The medical community refuses to use the word addiction because if sugar is addictive then the food industry has been selling an addictive substance to children for fifty years.

He says it anyway. That takes courage.

Tim Noakes has been a hero of mine for decades.

He is South African. Like me. He was an athlete. Like me. He wrote The Lore of Running, one of the definitive texts in sports science. He trained and competed and understood what it meant to push a body to its limits.

And then his own body broke. Type 2 diabetes. One of the fittest researchers in his field, eating exactly what his own research said he should eat. And his body said no.

He did what I did. He investigated and he discovered that carbohydrate intolerance is individual, that many people including elite athletes cannot metabolize carbohydrates without metabolic damage, and that the high-carb diet he had spent his career recommending was destroying the people who trusted him.

So he changed his position. Publicly. And the South African medical establishment put him on trial. Professional misconduct. For telling people to eat differently.

The trial lasted years. He was found not guilty. He kept going.

If you remember the Atkins diet, Atkins was demonized for saying meat was not the enemy. They went after him and they discredited him for saying that humans should eat the food humans have eaten for millions of years. Tim Noakes picked up that fight and built the scientific foundation underneath it. The Banting diet. The real food movement. The courage to say that the dietary fat-heart hypothesis was the greatest scientific fraud of the twentieth century.

When I found Tim Noakes, I did not just find a scientist. I found a South African who had walked the same path I was walking. An athlete whose body had been betrayed by the same dietary advice. A man who had been told he was wrong by the same establishment and refused to stop telling the truth.

These people are giants. Nina Teicholz, Philip Ovadia, Aseem Malhotra, Robert Cywes, Tim Noakes. And there are more. Stephen Sinatra, William Davis, James Roberts. Warriors who started this movement and continue to fight for it.

I am not a doctor. I am not a scientist. I am a citizen scientist standing on the shoulders of these people. They gave me the knowledge and the courage and the hope that I could survive.

Four of them became my co-founders. Because when I showed them my story, they saw every patient they had ever failed to reach in time. A man who almost died because the system was designed to sell pills, not find truth. My story was not unique to them. My story was proof that the system they had been fighting against for years was still winning. Still missing the root causes. Still prescribing the same drug. Still asking patients who are you to question this.

They said yes to building something together. Not because of a business plan. Because the mission was personal. For all of us.

CHAPTER 12

THE INVESTIGATION

ONCE I FOUND THE DOCTORS AND THE SCIENCE AND THE HOPE, I did what any person with a tennis player's stubbornness and nothing left to lose would do.

I ran every test my cardiologist never ordered.

Not some of them. All of them. Every marker I had read about at 2 AM on forums, every test that the survivors on Facebook said changed their understanding, every biomarker that the doctors who left the system said mattered more than cholesterol.

I turned myself into a laboratory. And what I found made me furious.

My cardiologist had been watching one number for fourteen years. LDL cholesterol. He had built my entire treatment plan around lowering that number, prescribed me three different drugs to crush it, and told me I would die without those drugs. When I brought him a peer-reviewed study suggesting there might be other factors, he asked me who I was to question the science.

Here is what the science actually showed when someone finally looked.

My fasting insulin was 8.5. Optimal is 2 to 5. I was nearly double the high end of functional optimal. My pancreas was working overtime to keep my blood sugar in range, and this is what insulin resistance looks like in its earliest stages, the thing that Joseph

Kraft showed in 14,384 patients in 1975 shows up decades before diabetes, decades before a heart attack. A $30 test. Never ordered.

My HOMA-IR was elevated, the gold standard calculation for insulin resistance. You take your fasting insulin and your fasting glucose and you run a simple formula. Optimal is under 1.0. Mine was well above that. The metabolic condition that Gerald Reaven identified at Stanford in 1988 as the root of metabolic syndrome. The numbers were sitting in the same blood draw. Nobody did the math.

My hs-CRP was 3.2. High-sensitivity C-reactive protein. A direct measure of systemic inflammation and one of the strongest independent predictors of cardiovascular events. Optimal is under 0.5. I was at 3.2. My body was on fire from the inside, chronic low-grade inflammation damaging my arteries every single day. Never tested until I asked for it myself.

My TSH was flagged high in four of seven panels. My thyroid had been underperforming for over a decade, the organ that regulates metabolism, energy, body temperature, and heart function was struggling, and nobody said a word. Four flags. Fourteen years. Zero conversations.

My triglycerides were 165, my HDL was 38, and my ratio was 4.3. Optimal is under 1.5. This ratio was sitting in the same lipid panel that my doctors used to prescribe statins. They saw the LDL and prescribed a drug. They did not calculate the ratio that actually mattered.

Homocysteine. Never tested. Vitamin D. Never tested. Two markers that directly impact cardiovascular risk. Simple blood tests available at any lab. Never ordered.

Then I tested my genes.

I was in a hotel room in El Paso, Texas, when I opened the email. I had sent my saliva in weeks earlier, a simple genetic test, spit in a tube and mail it and wait. And now the results were sitting in my inbox and I was afraid to open them.

The room was small and quiet. The air conditioner hummed against the window. I was sitting on the edge of the bed with my phone in my hand and my heart beating faster than it should have been for a man sitting still.

Getting your genetic results back is different from getting blood work. Blood work tells you where you are. Genetics tell you who you are. It is a scorecard that defines you. Not what you did wrong but what you were born with. What you cannot change. What you will carry for the rest of your life.

I opened the email. I saw the letters. APOE. Then the numbers. 3. That is good. Three is the common variant, the safe one. And then at the end, the number that changed everything.

4.

APOE e3/e4.

I sat in that hotel room and I felt doomed. APOE e4 is one of the most important genetic markers in medicine. It determines how your body processes cholesterol and fat. The e4 variant is associated with increased cardiovascular risk and a 40 percent higher risk of Alzheimer's disease. About 25 percent of the population carries at least one copy.

I carry one copy. And the first thing I thought was not about my heart. It was about my brain. I have the Alzheimer's gene. I am destined to lose my mind.

I sat there in El Paso with the air conditioner rattling and the parking lot lights coming through the curtains and I Googled APOE e3/e4 and all I found was fear. Stories of decline. Statistics about risk. The weight of a genetic inheritance I did not ask for and cannot return.

My brother did the test. He does not carry it. My sister did the test. She does not carry it. The gene skipped them and landed on me and then it passed through me to some of my children.

But here is what I know now that I did not know in that hotel room. APOE e4 is one of the oldest genetic variants in the human genome. We carried it for a reason. It helped us survive. Our bodies were not made to die. They were made to adapt. Millions and millions of years of evolution designed every gene in our body to serve a purpose, and APOE e4 was that purpose in a different world. A world without processed food. Without seed oils. Without Gatorade.

The diet I had been eating for thirty years, the pasta and the bread and the low-fat everything and the margarine, was the exact diet that the APOE e4 genotype processes poorly. I was eating the worst possible food for my specific genetics on the recommendation of doctors who never tested my genetics.

A hundred dollars. That is what an APOE test costs. One hundred dollars to know how your body handles fat, to know whether the dietary advice your doctor is giving you is helping or killing you. Nobody tested it. And I ate against my DNA for thirty years.

My son David carries the same variant. He is sixteen years old. But David knows. He found out at fifteen. Not in a hotel room filled with fear but at home, with a father who could explain what it means and what to do about it. That is the difference between knowledge and ignorance. Between a hundred dollar test and a lifetime of eating the wrong food.

Then came the result that almost broke me.

Lp(a). Lipoprotein little a. An inherited particle that increases clotting risk and promotes plaque formation. It does not respond to diet or exercise. It does not respond to statins. It is 100 percent genetic. You either have it or you do not.

I have it. And my number peaked at 276. That is high.

APOE e3/e4. 9p21 GG. And now Lp(a) at 276. Three genetic markers. Three loaded guns. All inherited. All permanent. All associated with cardiovascular disease.

I felt like my destiny was to die.

For someone with my personality, that feeling was unbearable. I am a problem solver. That is what tennis taught me. Every point is a problem and you deal with the weather and you deal with the opponent's forehand and you deal with not feeling well. You are constantly solving problems in real time. That is what made me a professional athlete and what made me successful in business.

But when someone tells you that you have three genetic risk factors and you look at the statistics on people who carry them, you go into a mode that the problem solver in you cannot fix. Fear mode. The feeling that no matter what you do, the genes will win.

And then the problem solver woke up.

Hold on. People have lived with these genetics for millions of years. Millions. Humans have carried APOE e4 and high Lp(a) since before recorded history. They found calcium in the arteries of mummies in pharaoh tombs in Egypt. Heart disease existed thousands of years ago, but those people were not eating Gatorade and margarine. They were not insulin resistant from orange juice. The disease existed, but the modern triggers, the ones that got me, are the ones we can control.

And here is the part that changed everything. Lp(a) is not a mistake. It is a feature. It is a clotting factor. When our ancestors were surviving on the plains and got cut or wounded, Lp(a) made their blood clot faster. It kept them alive. It was a survival advantage. The same molecule that modern medicine calls a risk factor was once the reason our species did not bleed out.

I tried niacin. It worked on the number. I brought my Lp(a) down from 276 to 52. A genetically determined marker that the medical establishment says cannot be moved. I moved it.

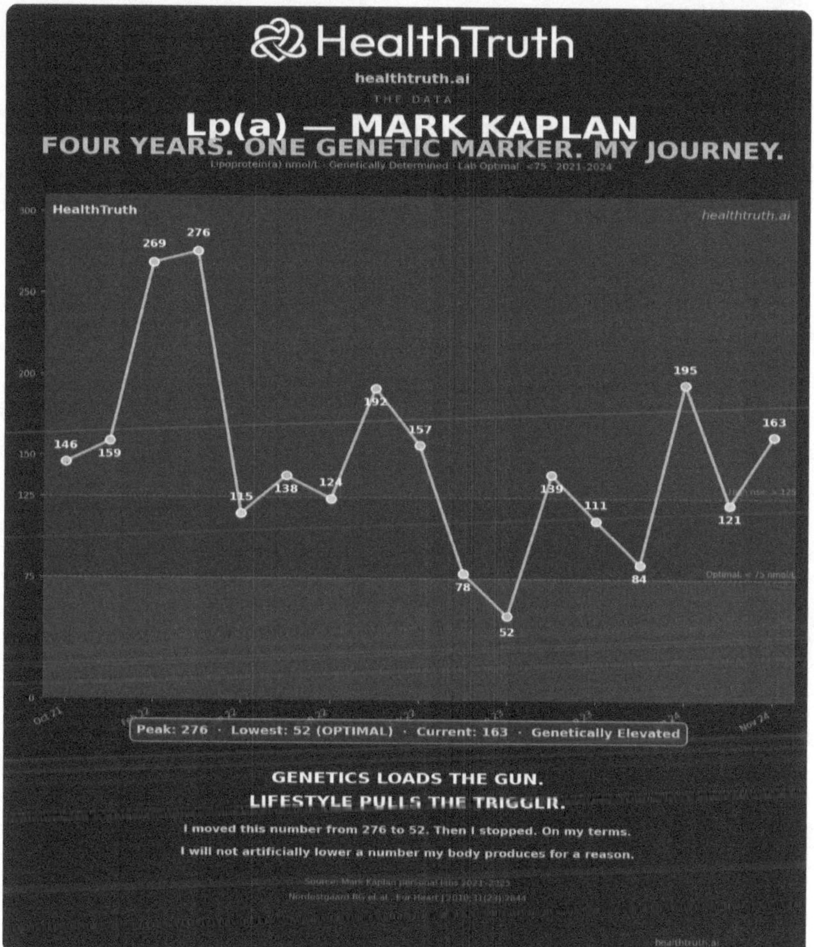

Mark Kaplan personal labs, 2021–2025. Reference: Nordestgaard BG et al., European Heart Journal, 2010;31(23):2844.

But then my liver enzymes shot up. AST and ALT, the markers that tell you your liver is under stress. My body was telling me something. It was telling me to stop.

So I stopped.

I am not going to artificially lower a number that is hurting my body to lower. That is exactly what statins do. Find a number, build a drug, push it down, ignore the damage. I refused to do that with LDL. I will not do it with Lp(a) either.

And now I need to warn you about what is coming next. Because the pharmaceutical industry has seen the same number I have seen. And they see something different in it.

They see a market.

Right now, in 2026, multiple pharmaceutical companies are developing drugs to lower Lp(a). Novartis. Amgen. Others. They are spending billions. Clinical trials are underway. The press releases are starting. The medical conferences are buzzing. A new class of drugs is being built to do to Lp(a) exactly what they did to LDL.

Find a number. Build a drug. Market it with relative risk reduction. Get the FDA to approve it. Train the doctors. Write the guidelines. Prescribe it to millions.

I have seen this movie before. I lived inside this movie for two years while my cardiologist crushed my LDL to 40 with a drug that stole my memory and my personality and my will to live. I know the script. And the script is being rewritten right now with Lp(a) in the starring role.

Here is what they are not telling you.

Nobody knows if lowering Lp(a) with a drug will actually reduce heart disease. Nobody has proven it. The trials are measuring whether the drug lowers the number. That is not the same question as whether lowering the number saves lives. It was not the same question with LDL and it is not the same question with Lp(a).

Remember what happened with LDL. They built drugs that lowered the number beautifully. Statins crush LDL. Repatha crushes it even further. The number goes down. The press release writes itself. But 60 trials involving 323,950 people showed near zero mortality benefit. The FOURIER trial on Repatha showed 28 percent more cardiac deaths on the drug than on placebo. The number went down and people still died. Because the number was never the cause. The number was a bystander.

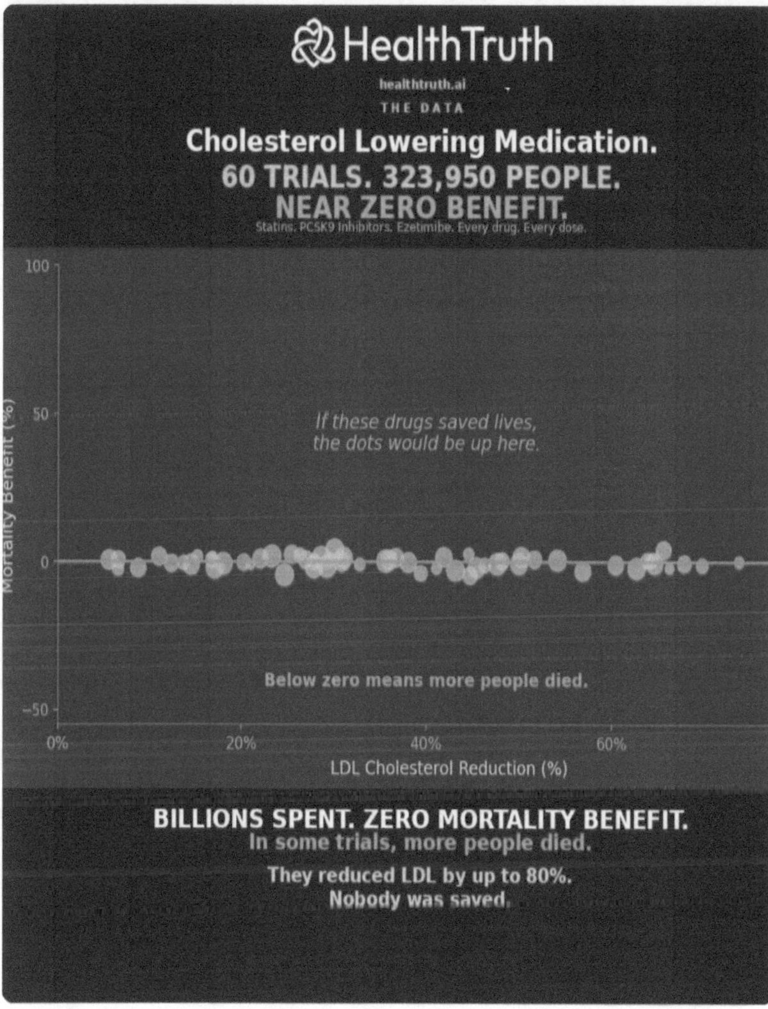

60 trials. 323,950 people. Pooled meta-analysis of statins, PCSK9 inhibitors, and ezetimibe trials.

Lp(a) is different from LDL in one important way. It is 100 percent genetic. You cannot change it with diet or exercise. It is inherited. And that makes it a more honest marker than LDL because it tells you something real about your biology. I believe everyone should know their Lp(a) number. Test it once. It does not change. Know what you are carrying.

But knowing your number is not the same as taking a drug to change it.

My Lp(a) peaked at 276. I tried niacin and brought it to 52. My liver said stop. I stopped. I did not override my biology to chase a number. Instead I managed every root cause that makes elevated Lp(a) dangerous. My insulin is optimal. My inflammation is low. My diet matches my genetics. My thyroid is addressed. The context around the Lp(a) is managed.

The pharmaceutical approach will be different. The pharmaceutical approach will be: your Lp(a) is high, take this drug, lower the number, do not ask questions about the eleven other things driving your disease. It will be the statin playbook all over again. One number. One drug. One hundred billion dollars.

If you just got your Lp(a) results and you are scared, I understand. I sat in a hotel room in El Paso and felt doomed when I saw my number. But before you take the drug they are about to sell you, ask yourself this question.

Did they test your fasting insulin? Did they check your hs-CRP? Did they look at your thyroid? Did they calculate your triglyceride-to-HDL ratio? Did they test your APOE genotype? Did they look at your homocysteine? Did they order a calcium scan?

If they tested one number and prescribed one drug, you are living my story. The same story. The same system. The same playbook. Just a different molecule and a different pill.

Do not let them do to Lp(a) what they did to LDL. Test it. Know your number. But fix the root causes first. That is how you manage Lp(a). Not with the next pill.

I believe in epigenetics. Genetics loads the gun. Lifestyle pulls the trigger. My Lp(a) is the loaded gun. It has been loaded for millions of years. My ancestors carried it and it kept them alive by clotting their blood when they were wounded on the plains of Africa. My body produces it for a reason.

My job is not to override my liver to chase a number. My job is to remove every trigger. I eat an ancestral diet the way my ancestors ate. Meat, eggs, fish, real food. No seed oils, no processed carbohydrates, no industrial foods that trigger the genes my body was never designed to encounter. My insulin is optimal, my inflammation is low, my diet matches my genetics, my thyroid is addressed. The root causes that make Lp(a) dangerous are managed. The gun is loaded, but I have removed every trigger I can find and I trust that a body running on the right fuel can manage what it was built to carry.

That is the insight that brought me back from the edge. You cannot change your genes, but you can change everything around them. Not by fighting your genetics. By honoring them.

And here is what you need to know about what is coming next. The pharmaceutical industry is already developing drugs to lower Lp(a). They see the same marker I see, but they see a market. A new number to medicate. A new drug to sell. The same playbook they ran with LDL cholesterol for forty years. But nobody knows if lowering Lp(a) with a drug will actually reduce heart disease. Nobody has proven it. They are building the drug before they have the evidence, the same way they built statins before they understood that LDL at 110 was not the problem.

Do not let them do to Lp(a) what they did to LDL. Test it. Know your number. But fix the root causes first. That is how you manage Lp(a). Not with the next pill.

Let me put this all in one place.

When I was on the operating table at 52, my body was dealing with twelve separate problems simultaneously. Not one. Twelve. Insulin resistance, chronic inflammation, thyroid dysfunction, genetic predisposition through APOE e4 and 9p21 GG, elevated Lp(a), a diet mismatched to my genetics, hormonal decline, vitamin D deficiency, gut dysfunction, elevated homocysteine risk, and triglyceride-to-HDL imbalance.

Twelve heads. One dragon.

My cardiologist saw one. Cholesterol. He prescribed one drug, a statin, and told me that one drug was the difference between life and death. He was looking at a dragon with twelve heads and trying to kill it by cutting off one. The weakest one. While the other eleven kept growing.

That is not a failure of one doctor. That is a failure of a system. A system that trains doctors to see one number, to prescribe one drug, to manage one symptom while the root causes multiply and compound and eventually put a 52-year-old tennis player on an operating table.

The system watched me for fourteen years. It had seven blood panels. It had more than enough data to find at least half of these problems before they combined to stop my heart.

It found none of them.

Because it was not looking.

CHAPTER 13

THE REVERSAL

I AM GOING TO SHOW YOU WHAT HAPPENED TO MY BODY WHEN I stopped listening to the system and started listening to the science.

These are not theories. These are not opinions. These are lab results. My lab results. Drawn from my blood. Measured in a laboratory. Compared over six years. Every number I am about to share is documented. You can verify them. That is the point.

When I had my heart attack at 52, here is what my body looked like from the inside.

My fasting insulin was 8.5. The earliest warning sign of metabolic dysfunction. A $30 test that was never ordered.

My triglycerides were 165. My HDL was 38. If you divide the first number by the second, you get a ratio of 4.3. That ratio is one of the strongest predictors of cardiovascular disease ever studied. Gaziano published this in 1997. Optimal is under 1.5. I was at 4.3. Nobody calculated it. Nobody mentioned it. It was sitting right there in the same blood panel they used to flag my LDL.

My hs-CRP was 3.2. Systemic inflammation. Screaming. Nobody tested it until I asked.

My testosterone was 506. Not clinically low, but for a lifelong competitive athlete, not where it should be. A sign that something deeper was wrong. Hormones do not exist in isolation. When your metabolic health deteriorates, your hormones follow.

My body fat was 24 percent. I weighed 198 pounds. I looked fine. I was active, but under the surface I was carrying visceral fat that was driving insulin resistance, inflammation, and hormonal dysfunction simultaneously.

My A1c was creeping toward pre-diabetic range. Candida. Gut issues. Thyroid dysfunction that had been flagged and ignored for years.

I was metabolically broken and every marker that mattered had been ignored while my cardiologist chased one number with a drug I could not tolerate.

That was before.

Here is after.

I changed what I ate. I stopped eating against my DNA. No more pasta. No more bread. No more margarine. No more low-fat yogurt. No more whole wheat toast. No more Gatorade. No more seed oils. No more of the foods that the government food pyramid and every doctor I had ever seen told me were healthy.

I replaced them with the foods they told me would kill me.

Meat. Eggs. Fish. Butter. Olive oil. Avocados. Nuts. Vegetables. Real food. Food with one ingredient. Food my great-grandmother would have recognized. Food that humans ate for 300,000 years before the food industry existed.

I addressed my thyroid. I ran more than 50 markers. I tested my genes. I worked with doctors who looked at the whole picture instead of one number.

And my body did something that my cardiologist said was impossible.

It healed.

My fasting insulin went from 8.5 to 2.5.

That single number tells you more about what happened inside my body than anything else on this page. My pancreas went from working overtime to barely having to work at all. The insulin resistance that had been building silently for decades. Gone. Not managed. Not medicated. Reversed. Through food.

My HOMA-IR, the gold standard measure of insulin resistance, dropped to 0.80. Optimal is under 1.0. I am not just in range. I am in the range that most 25-year-olds would be happy with.

My triglycerides went from 165 to 58.

My HDL went from 38 to 78.

My triglyceride-to-HDL ratio went from 4.3 to 0.74. From catastrophic to optimal. Not with a drug. With food.

My hs-CRP went from 3.2 to 0.8. The inflammation that the JUPITER trial taught me about. The marker my cardiologist never tested. It dropped by 75 percent.

My testosterone went from 506 to 851. No testosterone replacement therapy. No injections. No patches. No drugs of any kind. My body's own hormonal system recovered when the metabolic dysfunction that was suppressing it was removed. Imagine that. Fix the root cause and the symptoms resolve on their own.

My Lp(a) is genetically elevated. It always will be. I tried niacin and brought it from 276 to 52. Then my liver enzymes climbed and my body told me to stop. So I stopped. I do not chase numbers. I manage root causes. My insulin is optimal. My inflammation is low. My diet matches my genetics. The context around the Lp(a) is managed. I will not artificially lower a number my body produces for a reason. That is what statins do. I will not make the same mistake twice.

My body fat went from 24 percent to 12 percent. My weight went from 198 to 170 pounds. I weigh what I weighed in college at UC Irvine when I was on a tennis scholarship.

I am 58 years old.

My metabolic age is 43.

Zero medications. Not one pill. Not a statin. Not an aspirin. Not a blood pressure drug. Not a thyroid medication. Nothing.

Zero cardiac events in six years.

I still play competitive tennis. The sport that almost killed me is now proof that I fixed what the system missed.

Now here is the part that should make you angry.

My total cholesterol went from 210 to 262. It went up.

My LDL went from 130 to 168. It went up.

The number that my cardiologist spent years trying to crush to 40. The number that 92 million Americans take a pill every day to lower. The number that the entire pharmaceutical-cardiovascular complex is built on.

It went up and I got healthier than I have ever been in my life.

My cholesterol went up because I was eating the foods my body was designed to eat. My liver was producing the cholesterol it needed to build hormones, repair cells, and support brain function. Cholesterol is not poison. Your body manufactures it on purpose. Every single day.

The number went up. Every other marker improved. My risk went down. My inflammation dropped. My insulin normalized. My body fat halved. My energy came back. My memory came back. My creativity came back. My life came back.

If LDL cholesterol was the driver of heart disease, then a man whose LDL went from 130 to 168 should be dead. I am not dead. I am the healthiest I have been since my twenties and I have the bloodwork to prove it.

I want to be clear about something. I am not telling you to stop your medication. I am not a doctor. I am a citizen scientist. A patient. A heart attack survivor who decided to investigate why the treatment was worse than the disease.

What I am telling you is that the markers your doctor is watching may not be the markers that matter. What I am telling you is that there is a set of tests, most of them under $100, that paint a completely different picture of your cardiovascular health than a standard lipid panel. What I am telling you is that the food you eat, matched to your genetics, may be more powerful than any drug ever invented.

I know this because I am living proof.

Fasting insulin: 8.5 to 2.5. Triglycerides: 165 to 58. HDL: 38 to 78. hs-CRP: 3.2 to 0.8. Testosterone: 506 to 851. Body fat: 24% to 12%. Weight: 198 to 170. Lp(a): genetically elevated, managed through root cause, not drugs. Medications: multiple to zero.

Those are not opinions. Those are numbers. My numbers. Measured in a lab. Over six years.

The system said I would die without the drug.

The science said the drug was never the answer.

My body proved which one was right.

But the reversal was not just physical.

I remember the moment Melanie saw me come back. Not the numbers. Not the weight loss. Not the labs. The real me.

I had been on calls with the survivors I had found on forums, the tribe, the people who understood what a heart attack does to your mind. And after one of those calls, I put the phone down and walked into the kitchen where Melanie was making dinner and the kids were somewhere in the house and I sat down at the counter and I said something I had never said before.

Mel. I found my purpose. I want to help people.

Not: I think I am going to survive. Not: my numbers are improving. Not: I feel better. I want to help people. That was the sentence and she looked at me and she knew.

She told me later what she saw. She said: Mark, that was the moment I noticed everything changed. You were not about worrying about yourself dying every five minutes. You were about helping people. That was the change.

And she was right because once I started responding to people online. Once I started having conversations about what I went through. Once I started thinking about someone else instead of myself. I forgot about my own problems. I stopped checking my pulse. I stopped counting my breaths. I stopped planning my funeral.

The fear did not go away because my labs improved. The fear went away because I found purpose. When I was helping someone else survive what I had survived, I was not thinking about dying. I was thinking about living and that shift, from fear to purpose, healed something that no blood test can measure.

Melanie married a man who proposed after two and a half weeks because he saw what he wanted and went after it. She watched that man disappear into a fog of statins and fear and depression. And then she watched him come back. Not because of a drug. Not because of a doctor because he found a reason to fight that was bigger than his own survival.

Mark was back.

And then the anger came.

Once I stopped focusing on myself. Once the fear of dying every five seconds lifted. Once I started helping people on the forums and feeling the purpose flow through me. Something else arrived. Something I had not expected.

Rage.

How come? How come all these doctors and all these health professionals who are supposed to give us the guidelines and tell us what to do to heal were not doing it? How come years of checkups missed every root cause? How come a $100 genetic test that would have changed my life was never ordered? How come 92 million Americans are taking a statin and nobody is testing their fasting insulin? How come the system that is supposed to keep us alive is the system that almost killed me?

The hope that had saved me turned to fuel and the fuel ignited something that I recognized. Something I had not felt since the tennis court.

The underdog.

It felt like a tennis match. I had lost the first set. That was the heart attack. The statins. The Repatha needle. The will. The darkest period of my life. First set gone.

And now I was down 4-1 in the second set. That was the fear. The forums at 2 AM. The months of not knowing if I would survive. Down two breaks. Most people pack it in at 4-1 down in the second set after losing the first.

But I was coming back.

The healing was the comeback. Every pound I lost. Every marker that improved. Every night I spent on the forums finding Carl and Patrick and Fred. Every call with Philip. Every page of Nina's book. I was clawing back. Point by point. Game by game. 4-2. 4-3. 4-4.

And at 4-4, I made a decision. I am going to build something. I am going to go up against pharmaceutical companies if I have to. I am going to tell people the truth. I am going to show them the studies. I am going to prove that what the system told them was a lie and nothing is going to stop me.

Because you know what is behind me? The truth. The truth is behind me and behind every patient who has been drugged and not tested. Every person sitting in a doctor's office being told their cholesterol is the problem when their insulin is on fire. Every parent feeding their children margarine because the guidelines said so. The truth is behind all of us and the truth does not lose.

I started building. I reached out to Philip. To Rob Cywes. To Aseem. To Noakes. I told them what I wanted to create. A medical platform. A root cause platform. An AI that could take everything I had spent six years learning and deliver it to any patient on the planet in minutes. Not in 14 years of missed tests. In minutes.

The vision of HealthTruth | Neo came from that anger. Not from a business plan. Not from a market opportunity. From a man who had been down 4-1 in the second set and decided to fight his way back. The same way he had fought his way from the bottom of a college tennis team to a trophy from Arthur Ashe. The same way he had walked on with no scholarship and beaten the number one team in the country.

The underdog was back and this time, the match was bigger than tennis.

PART FOUR

THE MISSION

FROM PATIENT TO ADVOCATE.
FROM CITIZEN SCIENTIST TO CEO.
FROM SURVIVAL TO MOVEMENT.

CHAPTER 14

THE THREAD THAT CHANGED EVERYTHING

I HAD NO EXPERIENCE DOING THIS.

I had never posted on social media about my health. I had never written publicly about my heart attack. I had never told strangers about the statins or the depression or Sarah sitting me down in the living room. For five years, everything I had learned, everything I had survived, lived inside my family and the small tribe of survivors I had found on Facebook forums at 2 AM.

Then one day, a few months ago, I decided to go public.

I set up an account on X. I sat down at my kitchen table and I wrote something from my heart. Not a strategy. Not a content plan. Not a thread optimized for engagement. Just the truth. My story. The heart attack. The statin nightmare. The daughter. The firing. The reversal. The numbers. All of it. Laid out the way I would tell it to a friend at dinner.

I posted it and I went to bed.

The next morning I put my Apple Watch on.

It would not stop.

Every second. Beeping. Vibrating. Notifications. Likes. Follows. Replies. Messages. Signups. It did not stop. Not for an hour. Not for a day. For two full days my wrist would not stop buzzing.

I was flying to Miami the next day. I got on the plane. Same thing. The entire flight. My phone lighting up. My watch pulsing. Strangers finding my story and responding to it with a force I had never experienced.

By the time I landed, 3,000 people had signed up to the HealthTruth | Neo waitlist. 4,000 people had followed me on X. My story had reached over 800,000 readers.

I had no publicist. No advertising budget. No media contacts. No content team. Just a guy from Johannesburg who had a heart attack and told the truth about it.

Eight hundred thousand people stopped their day to read what happened to me.

I was blown away, but I was not surprised.

I had spent years on Facebook forums. I knew these people existed. I knew they were scared. I knew they were on statins and questioning them. I knew they had thyroid flags that had been ignored and insulin levels that had never been tested. I knew they were lying awake at 2 AM the same way I had, searching for proof that they were going to survive.

I just did not know how many of them there were.

The messages came in waves and they all said the same thing.

> *This is my story.*
> *My doctor never told me this.*
> *I wish I knew this sooner.*
> *I am 54 and this could have been me.*
> *My husband died last year. He was on a statin. Nobody tested anything else.*

Men in their 50s who had just been put on statins and were terrified. Women whose husbands had had heart attacks and wanted to know what tests to ask for. People sharing their own lab numbers in the replies. Their TSH. Their fasting insulin. Their triglyceride-to-HDL ratios. Asking me to look at them. Sending photos of lab reports with numbers circled and arrows pointing to the flags their doctors had ignored.

I felt an enormous amount of responsibility. These were not followers. These were patients. People in pain. People trapped in the same matrix I had been trapped in and they were reaching out to a stranger on the internet because the system they were paying to help them had failed.

I knew I was on the right path and I knew I had to make it more powerful.

That is when I figured out the charts.

The studies that changed my life were published in medical journals. The Women's Health Study. The Sachdeva study. The JUPITER trial. The FOURIER trial. Peer-reviewed. Rigorous. Transformative and completely unreadable for a normal person.

Pharma knows this. They publish 20-page studies filled with statistical jargon and confidence intervals and p-values. No 75-year-old woman is going to read a 20-page study. No 55-year-old man who just got put on a statin is going to download a PDF from JAMA Cardiology and parse the methodology section. That is the point. The studies exist. The data is there, but it is locked behind a wall of complexity that only doctors can climb and the doctors are being trained by the pharmaceutical companies.

So I started translating.

I took the most important studies in cardiovascular medicine and turned them into charts that a five-year-old could understand. Bar charts. Simple colors. Big numbers. One finding per image.

Statins work for 1 out of 100 people. The other 99 get side effects with no benefit. I made a bar chart. One green bar. Ninety-nine red bars. A child could look at that chart and understand the math that pharmaceutical companies spend billions obscuring.

The Women's Health Study. Diabetes is a 10x risk factor. Cholesterol is 1.4x. I made a bar chart. Two bars. One ten times taller than the other. The tall one is what they never test. The short one is what they medicate. A child could see the absurdity.

136,905 patients hospitalized with heart attacks. 75 percent had normal cholesterol. I made a chart. Three quarters of the bar in one color. Normal cholesterol. Heart attack anyway. That one image did more than a thousand words of explanation.

I attached these charts to my threads. Study name. Journal. Year. Sample size and a visual that made the finding undeniable.

They went viral. Immediately. People were screenshotting the charts and sending them to their doctors. Saving them to show their spouses. Printing them out and bringing them to appointments. The charts became the evidence that patients had never been given. The translation of science into truth that anyone could see.

I had found the weapon. Not anger. Not argument. Clarity. Simple, visual, cited clarity that made the pharmaceutical narrative impossible to defend.

The threads kept coming. Each one reaching hundreds of thousands of people.

The blood work thread. Twelve years of my actual lab results. Year by year. Panel by panel. Every LDL flag. Every ignored TSH. The repetition of "FLAGGED HIGH" over and over until the reader is furious on my behalf. 483,000 views. People calling it the most transparent thing they had ever seen from a patient because nobody does that. Nobody posts their actual medical records on the internet and walks you through what was missed.

The Alzheimer's thread. My APOE e3/e4 gene. The connection between insulin resistance and brain disease. Suzanne de la Monte at Brown calling Alzheimer's Type 3 diabetes. 761,000 views.

The statin thread. Seventeen posts. Every study cited with author, journal, year, and sample size. The absolute risk reduction. The FOURIER trial where LDL was crushed to 30 and more people died on the drug.

In three weeks, my following went from a few hundred to over 14,000. The HealthTruth | Neo waitlist passed 4,000. Without a single dollar of paid advertising.

In the first two months alone, the numbers were staggering. 11.1 million impressions. 76,000 likes. 47,000 bookmarks. 20,000 retweets. Over 17,000 followers. From zero. No paid ads. No promotions. Just the truth.

47,000 people saved our content to come back to later. That is the deepest form of engagement on X. People are building personal libraries of this science. Posts hitting 500,000 to 900,000 views with no advertising. The movement is real. People are waking up.

Bill Ackman, the investor, shared my Alzheimer's thread with his audience of over a million followers. Not because I asked him to because the science resonated. Prof. Tim Noakes was engaging in the replies. Confirming the data. Adding his own perspective. A globally respected scientist publicly backing the claims of a citizen scientist.

The statin debate drove more engagement than any other topic. Every time I posted about statins, the replies split into two camps. People who had experienced what I experienced and doctors who defended the guidelines. Both camps drove impressions. Both camps drove reach. The defenders thought they were discrediting me. They were amplifying me.

I learned something in those weeks that I carry with me every day.

The most powerful content in the world is not a study. It is not a chart. It is not a doctor's credential. It is a person standing in front of you saying: this happened to me. I almost died. The system failed me. Here are the numbers. Here is the proof and here is what I did about it.

My personal story post hit over 800,000 views. A thread about root cause science that started with a study instead of a personal detail got 8,000. Same account. Same audience. Same week. The difference was 100 to 1.

People do not share science. They share stories about people who were failed by the system and found a way out. They share those stories because they see themselves in them because they are scared because nobody has told them the truth.

But here is what I also realized. One man on X cannot do this alone. No matter how many threads I write. No matter how many charts I make. I cannot answer every question. I cannot review every lab panel. I cannot be available at 2 AM when someone is scared and Googling the same things I Googled five years ago.

These people do not just need information. They need an ecosystem. They need doctors who practice this type of medicine. They need communities of survivors. They need the charts and the studies in a format they can understand. They need someone to walk them across the chasm. Like a Grand Canyon between where they are and where they need to be.

Nobody is firing every doctor. People need doctors. Good doctors. Doctors who spend more than ten minutes. Doctors who test more than one number. Doctors who ask why before they prescribe what.

What I want to build is that ecosystem. Doctors. Survivors. Science. Community. AI. All of it connected. All of it working together. Not to replace the medical system. To complete it. To fill the gap that almost killed me and is still killing people every single day.

The threads were not the mission. The threads were proof that the mission needed to exist.

CHAPTER 15

THE DOCTORS WHO SAID YES

WHEN I FIRST IMAGINED BUILDING SOMETHING, I did not imagine a company. I imagined a solution to the hardest problem I had ever faced.

Because what I was doing as a patient was almost impossible.

I had to find the studies on YouTube. I had to find the books. Nina's book. Philip's book. I had to find the forums. William Davis's forum with 16 years of data. I had to find the people. Carl. Pat. Fred. I had to message them, email them, befriend them. I had to find the doctors. Philip. Aseem. Rob. Noakes. I had to find the vitamins. K2. Armour Thyroid. CoQ10. I had to fire my cardiologist. I had to order my own genetic tests. I had to read my own blood work because nobody would explain it to me.

It was like walking through a field of lies trying to find pieces of truth scattered across the internet. YouTube. Facebook forums. Amazon books. Podcast episodes. Medical journals I could barely understand. Every piece of the puzzle was somewhere different and nobody had put the puzzle together.

The medical system does not help these people. You go there for 10 minutes. They give you a drug. You go home. That is the system. Ten minutes. One number. One pill. Next patient.

And I thought: what if we built a platform?

What if a person with heart disease could come to one place. One website. Put their data in. Get a report. Have their blood work read by AI that understands root cause science. See what to eat for their genetics. Connect to doctors who practice this way. Watch the videos. Read the studies. Find the people who made it through. All in one place. Without spending six years at a dining room table at 2 AM trying to piece it together the way I did.

I started to build it in my head as I was going through the system as a patient. Every obstacle I hit became a feature. Every moment of frustration became a product requirement. I could not find my genetic data in one place. Feature. I could not connect to people with similar blood work. Feature. I could not get my doctor to explain my labs. Feature. I could not find the studies in a format I could understand. Feature.

The biggest strength I had was that I was the patient. I went through the system. I understood every nuance. The fear of dying. The confusion of the labs. The loneliness of the research. The hope of finding someone who survived. I understood the product because I was the user.

And here is what my 25 years in corporate marketing and insurance taught me. These functional medicine doctors have the truth. They are telling the truth. Their patients are getting better, but the truth is hidden. Every one of these doctors is a small voice. A shingle on a door. A practice in one city. They are like small voices in the wind and nobody can hear them.

Nobody has put a Cleveland Clinic brand around them. Nobody has put an Apple brand around them. Nobody has built the big tent. The big umbrella. The trust. The credibility. The platform that brings all of these voices together and amplifies them so that a scared patient at 2 AM can find the truth in minutes instead of months.

And I realized why nobody has built it because nobody makes money off this product. The sick care system makes money from drugs. From surgeries. From managing chronic disease forever. A platform that actually heals people is a product that no pharmaceutical company would ever fund. No hospital would ever build. No insurance company would ever promote.

So I would build it.

The truth is there. People are getting better. It is a great product. It just needs brand. It needs trust. It needs credibility. It needs doctors. It needs AI. It needs a founder who has been through the system and understands what patients need.

If you build it, they will come.

That was the genesis of HealthTruth | Neo.

But I am not a doctor and a platform full of science without doctors is a library. Useful but incomplete. People do not just need information. They need to trust the person giving it to them and in medicine, trust comes with credentials.

I needed doctors who understood what I had been through. Not doctors who would nod politely and recommend a statin. Doctors who had seen the same system failure and had the courage to say so out loud.

I already knew who they were. I had found them in the dark hole. Their books were the ones I read at 2 AM. Their lectures were the ones I watched on YouTube when my memory started coming back. Their studies were the ones I printed out and brought to a cardiologist who told me I was not qualified to read them.

So I reached out. One by one. A citizen scientist with no medical degree, no platform, and no funding. Asking four of the most respected voices in root cause medicine to build something with him.

I expected resistance. What I got was recognition.

Philip Ovadia was the first to understand.

He is a cardiac surgeon. He has spent his career cutting open chests. When I told him my story, he did not react the way most doctors would. He did not ask about my LDL. He did not suggest a different statin. He listened and when I finished, he said something I will never forget.

He said he had operated on me a thousand times.

Not me specifically, but me. The patient who ended up on his operating table because the system was watching the wrong numbers. The patient who could have been saved with a conversation about root cause but instead needed surgery.

He joined because he was tired of operating on people who should never have been on his table.

Aseem Malhotra had been publishing the evidence for years.

He had put his name on papers in the BMJ that challenged the statin consensus. He had endured the professional consequences of telling the truth in a system that punishes truth-tellers. When I told him about my cardiologist dismissing the JUPITER trial and asking "who are you to read these studies," he did not laugh. He recognized the pattern.

He had been that patient's advocate in medical journals. I was that patient standing in front of him.

Aseem joined because he had spent years writing papers that the medical establishment ignored. He wanted to build something that put the science directly in the hands of the people who needed it. Not filtered through pharmaceutical-funded guidelines. Not interpreted by a doctor with seven minutes and a statin prescription pad. Direct. Unfiltered. Patient-facing.

Robert Cywes saw something in my story that most people miss.

I told him about the 30 years of pasta and bread and Gatorade and low-fat everything. The foods I ate because the system told me they were healthy. The foods I could not stop eating even when I suspected they were not good for me. The way I would reach for bread without thinking. The way sugar was woven into every meal.

He called it what it was. Addiction.

I was not weak. I was not undisciplined. I was addicted to carbohydrates the same way an alcoholic is addicted to alcohol. The same neural pathways. The same reward cycle. The same inability to stop and the entire food industry was designed to keep me addicted because addicted people are repeat customers.

Robert joined because my story proved his thesis. A lifelong athlete eating the foods the system prescribed, unable to stop, developing metabolic disease, having a cardiac event. I was the case study for everything he had been teaching.

Tim Noakes understood me before I finished my first sentence.

When I told him I was from Johannesburg, something shifted. Two South Africans. Two men who grew up in the same country. Ate the same foods. Trusted the same science and both had their bodies break because of it.

When I told him about the Gatorade and the carb-loading and the performance diet that fueled my tennis career while destroying my metabolism, he nodded. He had recommended that exact diet to athletes for decades before his own body taught him he was wrong.

When I told him about being dismissed by my cardiologist for reading studies, he told me about being put on trial for changing his dietary recommendations. A formal hearing. Years of legal proceedings. His career and reputation on the line because he had the audacity to tell people that the dietary guidelines were wrong.

He was found not guilty and he kept going.

Tim joined because I was the patient version of his scientific journey. He had arrived at the truth through research. I had arrived at the truth through nearly dying. We were standing in the same place. Looking at the same broken system. From different sides.

None of them joined because of a business plan.

I did not have a pitch deck. I did not have revenue projections. I did not have a product mockup or a technology stack or a marketing strategy. I had my story. My lab results. My genetic data. My before and after numbers and a question.

Why does this not exist?

Why is there no place where a scared 52-year-old man can find root cause science, functional ranges, genetic context, and a community of survivors in one place? Why does the gap between what people need and what the system provides have to be this wide?

Four doctors. Four people who had spent their careers fighting the same system from different angles. A surgeon who was tired of operating too late. A cardiologist who was tired of publishing papers nobody read. A metabolic surgeon who was tired of treating the symptom instead of the addiction. A sports scientist who was tired of being punished for telling the truth.

They looked at my story and they saw every patient they had ever failed to reach in time. A man who almost died because the system did exactly what it was designed to do. Test one number. Prescribe one drug. Next patient.

They said yes.

Not to a company. Not to a product. To a mission.

Build the thing that should have existed before any of us needed it.

Four doctors. One citizen scientist. One mission.

The truth heals

CHAPTER 16

NEO

I NAMED THE AI AFTER THE CHARACTER who escaped the Matrix.

Not because I am a movie fan because it is the only metaphor that fits.

In The Matrix, everyone is plugged into a system that tells them reality is one thing while the truth is something else entirely. They eat what the system feeds them. They believe what the system tells them. They never question whether the world they see is the world that actually exists.

Then one person wakes up. Sees the truth and builds a way out for everyone else.

I lived inside a medical matrix for 20 years. My labs said "normal" while my body was metabolically failing. My doctors said "take a statin" while eleven root causes went undetected. My diet said "heart-healthy" while the foods I ate every day were mismatched to my DNA and driving me toward an operating table.

I woke up because my daughter told me the truth. I saw clearly because four doctors showed me the science and I built a way out because nobody should have to do what I did to survive.

The way out is called Neo.

Here is the problem that nobody has solved.

Ask ChatGPT a health question. You will get a competent answer. It will be accurate in a general sense. It will tell you to consult your doctor. It will present both sides. It will not take a position.

And it will be useless.

Because the person asking the question is not a medical professional. They do not know what to ask next. They do not know which follow-up matters. They do not know that the answer ChatGPT just gave them left out the three most important pieces of context for their specific situation.

ChatGPT requires you to be smart enough to ask the right question.

Neo only requires you to tap a button.

That is the difference. Not better AI. Not faster processing. Not a bigger database. A fundamentally different philosophy of how health intelligence should work.

A scared 55-year-old man just got told his cholesterol is high. His doctor wants to put him on a statin. He does not know what fasting insulin is. He does not know what APOE means. He does not know that 75 percent of heart attack patients have normal cholesterol. He does not know what to ask because nobody has ever told him what questions exist.

He opens Neo. He sees a button: "Should I really be taking a statin?"

He taps it.

Neo gives him an answer backed by science. Not both sides. The truth. What the pharmaceutical-funded trials show versus what the independent trials show. Where they conflict and why. What root cause markers his doctor should test before prescribing anything.

At the bottom of the response: a Key Insight card he can save. A Next Step card with a button that says "Take this step." He taps it.

Neo walks him through getting the right tests. What to ask for. What it costs. What the results mean. At the bottom: three follow-up questions he did not know to ask. He taps one.

Fifteen minutes later, he understands root cause metabolic health better than 90 percent of primary care doctors. He never typed a single word.

An 80-year-old grandmother can use this. A factory worker who has never heard of insulin resistance can use this. A teenager who just found out he carries the APOE e4 gene can use this.

The prompts are the product. The intelligence is the moat.

Neo is not one AI model. It is six.

Google Gemini. Anthropic Claude. OpenAI. xAI Grok. Meta Llama. Google Gemma. Six frontier AI models working together. Each selected for what it does best. When a better model launches anywhere in the world, Neo upgrades.

The intelligence is theirs. The medical brain is ours.

That medical brain is what makes Neo different from every other health AI on the planet. It is built on the positions of four doctors who staked their careers on root cause science. It uses a five-band system across 570 biomarkers calibrated to functional optimal ranges, not the disease-threshold ranges that the standard system uses. It classifies every study in its evidence base. Green: independent, peer-reviewed. Amber: mixed funding. Red: pharmaceutical-funded, excluded from primary recommendations. Blue: foundational science.

When Neo tells you that your fasting insulin of 18 is a problem even though your lab report says "normal," that is not a hallucination. That is four doctors and 30 years of independent research saying that the standard range allows a number that is three to four times higher than functional optimal and that the gap between "lab normal" and "actually healthy" is where disease forms.

That gap is where I lived for 14 years. That gap is where 88 percent of Americans live right now. That gap is what Neo was built to close.

Every response Neo gives follows the same architecture.

The Truth. What the science says. Not hedged. Not softened. Not "consult your doctor" as a way to avoid taking a position. The truth.

Key Insight. The one thing to remember. A card you can save or share. The thing you screenshot and bring to your next appointment.

Next Step. The one thing to do right now. A teal button: "Take this step." One tap and Neo walks you through it.

Go Deeper. Three follow-up questions you did not know to ask. Chevron arrows. Tap one and the investigation continues.

This is not a chat window. This is a guided investigation. The user never stares at a blank box wondering what to type. They follow a trail and the trail leads to the truth.

The seven pillars of root cause health are the investigation map.

Metabolic Health. The foundation. Insulin, blood sugar, metabolic syndrome.

Hormonal Health. The regulators. Thyroid, testosterone, cortisol.

Gut and Microbiome. The second brain. Digestion, absorption, immune signaling.

Inflammation and Immune. The fire. hs-CRP, cytokines, autoimmune drivers.

Toxic Load and Environment. The invisible burden. Seed oils, heavy metals, environmental exposures.

Stress, Sleep, and Nervous System. The recovery engine. HRV, cortisol rhythm, sleep architecture.

Nutrient Status. The raw materials. Vitamin D, magnesium, B12, omega-3.

General AI does not have a map. It answers whatever you ask. Neo has a map. It takes you where you need to go even when you do not know the destination.

I want to tell you about my children.

When my wife Melanie gave birth to our son David, in a birthing center, no drugs, the natural way she insisted on for all three of our children, I looked at him and I thought: I am done. Two girls and a boy. Sarah. Rebecca. David. Finished. Complete.

Having a son is something I cannot fully describe. A smaller version of yourself. The same stubbornness. The same optimism. The same way of attacking a tennis ball. David and I ski together. We travel the world. We play tennis on the same courts where my heart tried to stop. He wants to be a college player. Maybe a professional. He has the fight in him. I can see it.

When I had my heart attack, my whole family watched me fall apart. Sarah. Rebecca. David. Melanie. They watched the most positive, optimistic person they knew become negative, fearful, and convinced he was going to die. They lived through the statins. They lived through the depression. They lived through the will conversation and the midnight research and the firing.

And then they watched me come back.

David saw it all. He saw me before the change. Eating pizzas and drinking orange juice and following the same diet the system told everyone was healthy. He saw the heart attack. He saw the drugs. He saw the darkness and then he saw me change. He watched me lose 25 pounds. He watched me get strong. He watched me eat meat and eggs and the foods his father's doctors said would kill him. He watched my energy come back. My memory come back. My life come back.

And then David did something I did not ask him to do.

He switched.

But first I need to tell you about the genetic tests. I told all three of my kids they needed to test. David did it. Rebecca did it. Sarah did it.

The results came back. David: APOE e3/e4. The same variant that contributed to my heart attack. Rebecca: APOE e3/e4. The same.

When I saw those results on my phone, sitting at the kitchen table, I was initially sad. I thought: wow, they have the same condition I have. The same loaded gun. The same genetics that put me in a hospital bed at 52. My children are carrying it.

But then I felt hope because their destiny is not predetermined. They do not have the lack of knowledge I had. I did not know anything. I was eating everything the system told me to eat. My kids have knowledge and knowledge is power.

I sat David and Rebecca down. I said: look at how your dad is eating. Look at what happened. Look at the weight I lost. Look at how I feel. I lost 25 pounds. I was back to who I was. Positive. Strong. Alive.

I do not think they fully understood what the APOE number meant. It was just a number on a piece of paper, but they did not need to understand the number. They saw the changes in me. They saw how I was eating in the house. They saw the food on the table change and that changed everything.

There is no better way to influence your children than what you do. They watch you. They see everything.

David and I used to go to this place called Mario's. An Italian bakery. Pizza shop. We would sit there and eat pizzas together. Bread. Ice cream. All of it. That was our thing. Father and son at Mario's.

And then it stopped. I stopped going. I stopped ordering that food. When we went out, I ordered fish. I ordered steak. I stayed off the bread. David watched me not eat the food we used to eat together and he saw what happened to my body when I stopped.

David was 11. He was starting to put on some weight himself. He could see it and he saw the way I looked after the change. Lean. Strong. Fit. The father he remembered from before the heart attack and he just took it on.

Nobody told David to eat meat and eggs. Nobody forced him. He was on YouTube. He was on social media. He was reading. He was watching his father and one day, without any instruction from me, he switched. Meat. Eggs. Fish. Hardly any bread. Once in a while, but the pizzas at Mario's were done.

He was 11 years old when he made that choice. He is 16 now. He has been eating this way for almost five years.

My middle daughter Rebecca is at the University of Wisconsin. She carries the same APOE e3/e4. She eats no processed food. No bread. No junk. She made that change because she watched her father make it first.

My oldest daughter Sarah is at Ohio State. College is harder. The food environment is designed to make you eat the wrong things, but she sees the difference. She understands the science from everything I have shared on X and in our family conversations. She is moving toward a way of eating that matches her genetics. It is happening.

Three children. All watching their father nearly die. All watching him come back. All choosing, in their own time, in their own way, to unplug from the same food system that almost killed him.

That is what I am most proud of. Not the platform. Not the followers. Not the book. My children. Eating differently because they saw the truth play out in their own family.

David's cholesterol: optimal. His fasting insulin: optimal. His inflammation: undetectable.

Same genes as me. Different outcome.

Not because David is lucky because David has a father who almost died and refused to let the same thing happen to his son.

That is why I built this.

Not for the technology. Not for the business. Not for the followers or the waitlist or the threads that break a million views.

For the next David. The 16-year-old kid somewhere in the world right now who carries a genetic marker that nobody has tested. Who is eating the foods the system says are healthy while those foods are quietly mismatched to his DNA. Who will grow up and go to checkups and be told his cholesterol is the only number that matters. Who will take the statin if it gets high enough. Who will trust the system because why would you not trust the system.

Unless someone shows him the truth first.

That is what Neo does. That is what HealthTruth | Neo is. A way to see clearly before the crisis. A way to find the root cause before the root cause finds you. A way to unplug from a system that was never built to keep you healthy and plug into one that was.

Heart disease killed the generation before me. My father never had the information I have now. He trusted the system. The system did what the system does.

Heart disease nearly killed me. The system watched one number while every root cause went undetected because the food I ate for 30 years was mismatched to my DNA because nobody tested a $100 gene that would have changed everything.

Heart disease will not kill my children.

Not just David. All three of them. Sarah. Rebecca. David. They have all done their genetic testing. They are all putting their blood work in. They all know their APOE status. They all know how to eat for their genetics.

I did not have that information until I was 52 and lying in a hospital bed. My kids have it at 21, 19, and 16.

My brother and my sister did the same genetic tests. They do not carry the APOE e4 variant. They do not have the elevated Lp(a). The genes skipped them and landed on me and then they passed through me to some of my children. That is how genetics works. It is not a family-wide sentence. It is a loaded gun that gets handed to specific people and if nobody checks, nobody knows who is holding it.

My mother's family lived into their 90s in South Africa. My father's side died earlier, but not from heart disease. There was no obvious family history to raise a flag. No reason for any doctor to test my genes. No red line on a chart that said: this man needs to be watched differently.

But the genes were there. Silently. For 52 years. Waiting for the wrong diet and the wrong lifestyle to pull the trigger.

If I had been tested at 10 years old. If someone had looked at my DNA and said, Mark, you carry APOE e4 and elevated Lp(a), here is how you need to eat, here are the foods to avoid, here are the markers to watch. If that had happened, I would never have spent 30 years eating pasta and bread and Gatorade. I would never have developed insulin resistance. I would never have had chronic inflammation building silently in my arteries. I would never have had a heart attack at 52.

I believe HealthTruth | Neo is going to cure heart disease.

Not with a drug. Not with a surgery. With information. With a genetic test at 10 years old that tells you how your body works. With an AI that takes your genetics and your blood work and your lifestyle and tells you exactly what is loading the gun and exactly what will pull the trigger. With a platform that gives every human being on earth the knowledge to eat for their DNA before the damage starts.

That is not a fantasy. That is math. If you know which genes are loaded and you know which lifestyle factors pull the trigger, you can prevent the event. Not treat it after the fact. Not manage it with pills. Prevent it. Before it ever happens.

The current system cannot do this. Every specialty has its own silo. Cardiology looks at the heart. Endocrinology looks at hormones. Neurology looks at the brain. Gastroenterology looks at the gut. Nobody is putting all the systems together. Nobody is connecting the genetics to the diet to the inflammation to the thyroid to the insulin to the heart.

Except Neo.

My legacy is simple.

I want to give the next generation something I never had. A tool that tells them the truth about their body before their body has to tell them the hard way. A platform where a 10-year-old can put in their genetics and learn how to eat so they never end up on an operating table at 52.

I am not a doctor. I am a citizen scientist. A patient. A heart attack survivor who spent six years researching what went wrong and building the thing that should have existed before he needed it.

My father never had this information. He trusted the system. The system did what the system does.

I almost did not have this information. It took a heart attack, a statin nightmare, a daughter brave enough to tell me the truth, and six years of midnight research to find it.

My children have this information now. Sarah. Rebecca. David. They will never have to search for it in the dark.

And if I do this right, neither will yours.

I am 58 years old. My metabolic age is 43. Zero medications. Zero cardiac events in six years. I still play competitive tennis on the same courts where my heart tried to stop.

Genetics loads the gun. Lifestyle pulls the trigger and knowledge disarms them both.

The truth heals

EPILOGUE

A LETTER TO SARAH

Dear Sarah,

You were born in a birthing center. No drugs. Your mother and I lay with you between us in those first minutes. You were so small. We were so young and I remember thinking: I will spend the rest of my life protecting this person.

I got that backwards.

You have always been honest. From the time you could talk, you said exactly what you meant. No softening. No performance. Just the truth. You are spirited and courageous and you have never once been afraid to tell someone something they did not want to hear.

You are an old soul. You have always been beyond your years. I do not know where that comes from. Maybe it comes from watching your father compete on tennis courts around the world and learning that the people who win are the ones who refuse to pretend everything is fine when it is not.

When I had my heart attack and the drugs took me away from my family, you were the one who said what nobody else would say. Not because you were not afraid of hurting me because you were more afraid of losing me.

It takes courage to tell your father that he has changed. That he is not the same person. That the man sitting in front of you is not the man who raised you. You knew those words would hurt me. You said them anyway because you had already lost your father to the pills and the fear and the depression, and you were not willing to let that be the end of the story.

You did not give me a diagnosis. You did not hand me a study. You gave me something harder than that. You held up a mirror and showed me what I had become and then you trusted me to do something about it.

That moment in the living room changed the course of my life.

Everything I have built since then. The research. The doctors. The reversal. The platform. The book you are holding. All of it started because a daughter looked her father in the eyes and told him the truth.

I want to thank you for that. For your honesty. For your courage. For being willing to say the hard thing because you loved me too much to say the easy thing.

I want you to know that I am the happiest I have ever been. I wake up every day with gratitude. My mind is clear. My body is strong. I play tennis with your brother. I build things that help people. I live every day like it matters because you taught me that it does.

I owe my life to the doctors who showed me the science. I owe my health to the food that healed my body, but I owe my survival to you. You saved me by telling me the truth when the truth was the last thing I wanted to hear.

Rebecca and David and your mother Melanie have been with me through all of it. This family carried me when I could not carry myself, but it was you, Sarah, who changed the direction. You were the turning point.

Thank you for being honest with me. Thank you for being braver than I was. Thank you for refusing to let me disappear.

I love you.

Dad

The truth heals

AFTERWORD

THE OTHER SIDE

BY MARK KAPLAN, MAY 2026

I NEED TO TELL YOU WHERE I AM NOW. Not the numbers. You have seen the numbers. Not the platform. You have read about the platform. Where I am. The person. The man who spent Chapter 7 planning his funeral.

I am happy.

I know how strange that sounds after everything you just read. Sixteen chapters of fear and betrayal and fighting and midnight research and firing doctors and nearly losing my marriage and watching my children watch me disappear and the man at the end of all of it is telling you he is happy.

But that is the truth and this is a book about the truth.

I do not think about heart disease anymore. I do not think about dying. Not tomorrow. Not next week. Not at all. The fear that consumed every breath I took for months after my heart attack is gone. Not managed. Not suppressed. Gone. Replaced by something I did not expect and could not have predicted.

Gratitude.

I am grateful for my heart attack.

I know how that sounds. I almost did not write it, but it is true. I am grateful because the heart attack broke open a life that looked perfect but was quietly killing me. It broke open a medical system that I trusted blindly. It broke open a diet that I followed religiously. It broke open every assumption I had about health, about medicine, about what it means to take care of yourself.

And on the other side of all that breaking, I found something better than what I had before.

I found purpose.

I wake up every morning and I know exactly why I am here. I am here to help people who are where I was. Scared. Alone. Searching at 2 AM for proof that they are going to survive. I go on X and I reply to strangers who are asking the same questions I asked. I read their lab results and I point them toward the tests their doctors are not ordering. I tell them my story and I watch them realize they are not alone.

That gives me joy. Not satisfaction. Not a sense of duty. Joy. The kind that fills your chest and makes you want to do it again tomorrow.

I found people.

The doctors who became my co-founders are not just business partners. They are people who changed my life. Philip Ovadia. Aseem Malhotra. Robert Cywes. Tim Noakes. Nina Teicholz. These are human beings who risked their careers to tell the truth. Meeting them. Working with them. Building something with them. That is a gift the heart attack gave me.

I found health.

Real health. Not the fake health I had before, where I ate low-fat yogurt and passed my annual checkup and thought everything was fine. Real health that I can feel in my body every morning when I wake up.

Let me tell you what a day looks like now.

I wake up and I am grateful. That is the first feeling. Grateful to be here. Grateful that my energy is good. Grateful that the fog is gone and my mind is clear and my body works.

Most mornings I work out at home. Fifty minutes of cardio on my bike or my elliptical. Then I do my stretches. Some weights. It is convenient. I have everything I need in my house. When I am traveling, I do the same routine in the hotel gym. The routine does not change. The location changes. The commitment does not.

I have a far infrared sauna. Twenty-five minutes and if I am motivated, I jump in the ice bath. Some mornings I am. Some mornings I am not, but when I do it, I feel incredible. My body is awake. My mind is sharp. I am set up for the day.

Then I eat. Around 10 or 11 o'clock. Five or six eggs. All the yolks. We get these Amish organic eggs with the bright orange yolks. I eat them without guilt. Without fear. Without a single thought about cholesterol because I know what I know now.

I do not eat much for lunch. For dinner, around 5 or 6 o'clock, I sit down with my family. A piece of meat or fish. Low-carb vegetables. Water. Sparkling water. That is it. High protein. High fat. Almost no processed food. No bread. No seed oils. No orange juice. The food my body was designed to eat.

I play tennis. Singles with David when I am home. It pushes my heart. Builds collateral arteries. I play a doubles league with my friends. I cycle. I spend time with people I love.

My girls are back from college in the summer. Sarah and Rebecca. We are together. Melanie. The kids. Friends. Tennis. Family dinners. Life.

I am 58 years old. I weigh 170 pounds. The same weight I carried at UC Irvine when Arthur Ashe handed me that trophy. I play singles with my 16-year-old son who wants to go pro and I can keep up with him.

My mind is sharp. My memory is back. My creativity is back. The cotton wool is gone. The blank screen is gone. I think clearly. I move fast. I build things. I am more productive at 58 than I was at 48.

And I found something I did not know I was missing. The appreciation of time.

When you believe you are going to die, you stop living. I know that because I lived it. Every breath was a countdown. Every heartbeat was a warning. The future did not exist because I did not believe I would be there to see it.

Now I live the opposite way. I do not think too far ahead. I do not worry about things I cannot control. Nothing really bothers me because when you have been to the bottom. When you have sat in your living room and told your wife to get your will in order. When you have genuinely believed that Monday would be your last day on earth. After that, everything else is gravy.

I wake up every day and the first thing I feel is: I am alive.

Not as a thought. As a feeling. A physical sensation of gratitude that starts in my chest and spreads to my fingertips. I am here. I get another day. I get to see my kids. I get to play tennis. I get to build something that might help a stranger survive the same thing I survived.

That is the gift.

The heart attack did not just teach me about cholesterol and insulin and thyroid function. It taught me that every day is borrowed. That the life I was living before, the "perfect" life, the life where I never thought about dying, was actually a life where I never thought about living. I was on autopilot. Checking boxes. Following the plan. Never stopping to feel how extraordinary it is to simply be here.

I feel it now. Every single day.

Would I do it again? Would I go through the heart attack and the statins and the depression and the fear and the firing and the midnight research and the six years of fighting?

Yes.

Because the person I am today is someone I could not have become any other way. The people in my life. The purpose that drives me. The health I have earned through knowledge instead of luck. The joy I feel in ordinary moments that I used to take for granted.

I went from fear to joy. From no hope to absolute hope. From dying to living more fully than I ever have.

As dark as the place was, I am living in such light today.

And all I want to do is help you find that same light. That is why I built HealthTruth | Neo. That is why I wrote this book. I have other businesses. Other things I am involved with, but this is my passion. This is what gets me out of bed. The purpose of my life is to help as many people as I can reach the place where I am right now because five years ago I was in a very, very dark place and now I am here. With great energy. With family and friends. With my health.

And without health, you have no wealth. That is the truth.

If you are scared right now. If you just got a diagnosis. If your doctor handed you a bag of pills and told you this is your life now. If you are sitting at your kitchen table at 2 AM searching for proof that you are going to survive.

You are going to survive.

I am the proof.

And the truth heals

Continue the journey at neo.healthtruth.ai

MONDAY MORNING

I KNOW WHAT YOU ARE THINKING. You just read 16 chapters and an afterword and you are sitting there with a knot in your stomach because some of this sounded like your life. Your doctor said your cholesterol was high. You are on a statin. You have been feeling the fog. Or your husband is on a statin and he has not been himself. Or your mother just had a heart attack and she did everything right. Or you just got your blood work back and the only number they flagged was LDL.

You are where I was. And you are asking the same question I asked.

What do I do now?

Here is what you do. Monday morning. Not next month. Not when you get around to it. Monday.

You call your doctor's office and you ask for two tests. Just two. Fasting insulin and hs-CRP. You say those words exactly. Fasting insulin. hs-CRP. Write them down if you need to. Take this book with you if it helps.

These two tests cost under 60 dollars combined. They are available at any lab in the country. They do not require a specialist. They do not require a referral. They require a doctor who is willing to order them.

If your doctor says yes, you will have results in a few days. And those results will tell you more about your cardiovascular health than every cholesterol test you have ever taken combined.

A fasting insulin under 5 means your metabolic engine is clean. Your pancreas is not working overtime. The insulin resistance that drives heart disease, diabetes, and Alzheimer's is not forming. You are in a good place.

A fasting insulin above 8 means something is happening. Something that a standard blood panel does not show you. Something that a statin cannot fix. Something that your diet can.

An hs-CRP under 1.0 means your body is not on fire. The chronic inflammation that the JUPITER trial identified as a primary driver of heart disease is under control.

An hs-CRP above 2.0 means the fire is burning. And nobody lit a match to put it out because nobody checked the temperature.

Those two numbers are the beginning of seeing clearly. They are the first step out of the matrix. They are the difference between managing a number and finding the root cause.

Now here is the part nobody tells you.

If your doctor says no. If your doctor says those tests are unnecessary. If your doctor says your cholesterol is the only thing that matters and you should take the statin and come back in three months. If your doctor looks at you the way my cardiologist looked at me and says who are you to question this.

That tells you everything.

Not about the tests. About the doctor. A physician who refuses to order a 30 dollar insulin test for a patient who is asking for it is not practicing medicine. They are practicing the guidelines. And the guidelines were written by the system this book just showed you.

You do not need to fire your doctor that day. I am not telling you to do what I did. I am telling you to notice. Notice what happens when you ask. Notice whether your doctor is curious or defensive. Notice whether they want to investigate or dismiss. That reaction is data. And it is more valuable than any blood panel.

If they say yes, you are on your way. Bring the results to your next appointment. Ask what they mean. If your doctor does not know what functional optimal ranges are, bring this book. Show them the Protocol section. Or open Neo on your phone and let the AI walk both of you through it.

If they say no, find a doctor who says yes. They exist. Functional medicine doctors. Integrative cardiologists. Physicians who practice root cause medicine. They are out there. They are the Philip Ovadias and the Aseem Malhotras of the world. Small voices in the wind. But they are there. And Neo can help you find one.

Two tests. Under 60 dollars. One phone call on Monday morning.

That is where it starts. Not with a book. Not with a platform. Not with a thread on X. With you. In a doctor's office. Asking for the tests that my seven doctors never ordered in fourteen years.

The information that could have saved me exists today. It costs less than dinner. And nobody is ordering it.

Until you do.

And while you are waiting for Monday, do something tonight.

Go find your last blood panel. It is in a drawer or in your email or in your patient portal. Open it. Find two numbers. Triglycerides and HDL. They are on every standard lipid panel. Your doctor already has them.

Divide your triglycerides by your HDL.

If the answer is under 1.5, your lipid health is in a good place. If the answer is above 3.0, you have a problem that nobody mentioned to you because they were too busy looking at your LDL. That ratio was sitting in the same blood panel your doctor used to prescribe your statin. Nobody calculated it.

Mine was 4.3. Today it is 0.74. Same person. Different food.

You can do that math in thirty seconds. You do not need a doctor. You do not need a lab. You need a calculator and the blood work that is already sitting in your file.

Then on Monday, ask for the fasting insulin and the hs-CRP.

Then ask for one more thing. An Lp(a) test. Lipoprotein little a. You only need to test it once in your life because it is genetic. It does not change. It costs about 30 to 50 dollars. And it is the single strongest inherited risk factor for cardiovascular disease. I carry it. Arthur Ashe carried it. My children carry it. One in five people carry it and most of them do not know.

If your Lp(a) is normal, you can stop worrying about that piece. If it is elevated, you have information that could save your life and the lives of your children. Because if you carry it, they might too. That is how genetics works. The loaded gun gets passed down. And the only way to know who is holding it is to test.

My son David was tested at 15. He carries the same APOE e3/e4 and elevated Lp(a) that I carry. But David knows. He eats for his genetics. His markers are optimal. He will never have a heart attack at 52 wondering what happened.

That is the point of all of this. Not to scare you. To arm you. With tests that cost less than a pair of shoes. With information that the system has had for decades and never gave you. With the knowledge to walk into a doctor's office on Monday morning and say: I want to see the full picture. Not one number. The full picture.

And one more thing. While you are waiting for your results, change what is on your plate.

I am not going to tell you to follow a named diet. I am not going to say keto or carnivore or paleo or Mediterranean. I am going to give you one rule that is older than every diet book ever written.

Eat real food. Nothing in a package.

If it has a label with ingredients you cannot pronounce, do not eat it. If it has a health claim on the front of the box, be suspicious of what is inside the box. If it was made in a factory, your body was not made to process it.

Eat the food you would eat if you lived by the sea or on the land the way humans have lived for 300,000 years. Fish. Meat. Eggs. Vegetables that grow in the ground. Fruit that grows on a tree. Nuts. Seeds. Butter. Olive oil. Water.

Stop drinking your calories. No orange juice. No grapefruit juice. No soda. No sports drinks. I drank Gatorade on tennis courts for 30 years and it drove the insulin resistance that nearly killed me. Juice is sugar without the fiber. Your body does not know the difference between a glass of orange juice and a glass of soda. Your pancreas responds to both the same way.

If you look at the blue zones, the places on earth where people live the longest, they do not agree on whether to eat meat or fish or plants. But they all agree on one thing. They eat real food. Whole food. Food with one ingredient. Food their grandmothers would recognize. None of them are eating seed oils and low-fat yogurt and cereal from a box.

This is not about being perfect. This is about removing the things that are actively poisoning you. The seed oils. The processed carbohydrates. The sugar hiding in everything. Remove those three things and your body will start to tell you what it actually needs. Your hunger will regulate. Your cravings will quiet down. Your energy will stabilize.

You do not need a nutritionist for this. You need a grocery store with a perimeter. The real food is on the edges. The packaged food is in the middle. Stay on the edges.

Two tests on Monday. One ratio tonight. One genetic test that you only do once. Real food starting now.

That is your protocol for the next seven days.

The rest is in the pages that follow.

THE PROTOCOL

WHAT I DID

> *I am not a doctor. Nothing in this section is medical advice. This is what I did, personally, based on six years of research with four world-class doctors. Your genetics are different. Your markers are different. Your path will be different. Do not stop any medication or start any protocol without working with your healthcare provider.*

That said. Here is everything.

If I could go back 20 years and hand myself a piece of paper, it would be this list. These are the tests that would have caught what was building inside me a decade before the heart attack. Most of them cost less than a dinner out. None of them were ever ordered by any of my doctors.

Fasting Insulin—Cost: approximately $30. Available at any lab. No prescription needed in most states. This is the single most important test that the standard system does not order. It catches insulin resistance 10 to 15 years before blood sugar moves. My level was 8.5. Optimal is 2 to 5. Nobody tested it.

HOMA-IR—Calculated from your fasting insulin and fasting glucose. Your doctor can do the math or you can do it yourself. It is the gold standard measure of insulin resistance. Optimal is under 1.0. The standard system allows up to 2.5. That gap is where disease forms.

hs-CRP (High-Sensitivity C-Reactive Protein)—Cost: approximately $25. A direct measure of systemic inflammation. One of the strongest independent predictors of heart disease. Mine was 3.2. Optimal is under 0.5. The JUPITER trial proved this marker matters. My cardiologist never ordered it.

Full Thyroid Panel—Not just TSH. The full panel: TSH, Free T3, Free T4, Reverse T3, and thyroid antibodies. Cost: approximately $100 to $200 depending on the lab. My TSH was flagged HIGH in four of seven panels over 14 years. Nobody mentioned it. Functional optimal for TSH is 1.0 to 2.0. The standard system allows up to 4.5. That is not optimal. That is the threshold for disease.

Triglyceride-to-HDL Ratio—This is not a separate test. It is calculated from your standard lipid panel. Divide your triglycerides by your HDL. Optimal is under 1.5. Mine was 4.3. One of the strongest lipid predictors of cardiovascular disease. It was sitting in the same blood panel my doctors used to prescribe statins. Nobody calculated it.

Lp(a) (Lipoprotein little a)—Cost: approximately $30 to $50. A genetic lipoprotein. The single strongest inherited risk factor for cardiovascular disease. It does not respond to diet, exercise, or statins. You either have it or you do not. You only need to test it once in your life. Mine is elevated. Nobody tested it until I asked.

Homocysteine—Cost: approximately $30. An amino acid that at elevated levels damages the lining of blood vessels. Associated with increased clotting and cardiovascular events. Optimal is under 7. The standard system allows up to 15. Easily addressed with B vitamins if elevated.

Vitamin D—Cost: approximately $30 to $50. A hormone, not just a vitamin. Regulates immune function, inflammation, and cardiovascular health. Optimal is 50 to 80 ng/mL. The standard system calls 30 "sufficient." That is not sufficient. That is barely surviving. Most Americans are deficient.

HbA1c—Cost: approximately $20 to $30. A three-month average of your blood sugar. The standard system says 5.6 percent is "normal." Functional optimal is 4.6 to 5.2 percent. The gap between 5.2 and 5.6 is where pre-diabetes hides.

APOE Genotype—Cost: approximately $100. A one-time genetic test. Tells you how your body processes fat and cholesterol. APOE e4 carriers handle dietary carbohydrates and fats differently. The diet that is fine for an e3/e3 person can be metabolically destructive for an e4 carrier. I am e3/e4. I ate the wrong diet for my genetics for 30 years. One test would have changed everything.

9p21 Genotype—Cost: included in most genetic panels. The strongest genetic predictor of early heart attack. Does not cause disease on its own but tells you how vulnerable your arteries are to the damage caused by inflammation, insulin resistance, and a mismatched diet.

CAC Score (Coronary Artery Calcium)—Cost: approximately $100 to $200. Not a blood test. A low-dose CT scan that shows how much calcium has built up in your coronary arteries. A score of zero is extremely reassuring regardless of what your cholesterol says. A high score means the disease has been building. It is the closest thing to looking directly at your arteries without surgery.

The total cost of every blood test on this list is approximately $300 to $500. A standard lipid panel that leads to a statin prescription costs $25 and generates decades of recurring drug costs and follow-up visits.

One path finds the root cause. The other manages one number.

> *For a personalized test plan based on your age, genetics, and risk factors, ask Neo at neo.healthtruth.ai*

I do not follow a named diet. I am not carnivore. I am not keto. I am not paleo. I am not Mediterranean. I eat what my genetics and my blood work tell me to eat. The science decides. Not the tribe.

That said, here is what is on my plate today.

What I eat every day. Meat. Beef, lamb, chicken, turkey. Eggs. Usually three to four per day. Fish. Salmon, sardines, mackerel. The fattier the better. Butter. Real butter. Not margarine. Olive oil. Extra virgin. On everything. Avocados. Nuts. Macadamia, almonds, walnuts. Vegetables. Leafy greens, broccoli, cauliflower, asparagus. Berries. Blueberries, strawberries. In moderation.

What I removed completely. Seed oils. Soybean, canola, sunflower, safflower, corn oil. These are in everything. Every restaurant. Every packaged food. Every dressing. I avoid them like poison because for my genetics, they are. Processed food. Anything in a box with a health claim on the label. Bread. Pasta. Rice. Not because carbohydrates are evil for everyone. Because my APOE e4 genotype does not process them well. My blood work proved it. Sugar. In all forms. Refined, added, hidden. Gone. Margarine. The food that sat on my kitchen counter in Johannesburg for my entire childhood. Never again. Low-fat anything. If the fat has been removed, sugar has been added. That is how the food industry works. Gatorade. The drink that fueled my tennis career and my insulin resistance simultaneously.

How I think about food now. One ingredient. If my great-grandmother in Johannesburg would not recognize it, I do not eat it. Real food. Whole food. Food that humans ate for 300,000 years before the food industry told us to eat something different.

I do not count calories. I do not track macros obsessively. I eat until I am full. When you remove the processed carbohydrates and seed oils, your hunger signals start working again. You eat when you are hungry. You stop when you are not. It is the simplest thing in the world once the addictive foods are gone.

The result. I went from 198 pounds to 170. From 24 percent body fat to 12 percent. From a metabolic age of 58 to 43. Eating the foods my cardiologist told me would kill me.

> *For an eating plan matched to your specific genetics and blood work, ask Neo at neo.healthtruth.ai*

I take fewer supplements than most health influencers recommend. The HealthTruth | Neo rule is simple: test before you take. Do not guess what you are deficient in. Measure it. Then supplement only what your body actually needs.

My protocol was heavily influenced by the work of Dr. Steven Sinatra, a cardiologist who spent decades researching the metabolic causes of heart disease. His research on CoQ10 and mitochondrial energy production changed how I think about heart health.

CoQ10 (Coenzyme Q10)—This is the foundation of my heart protocol. Sinatra's research showed that CoQ10 is essential for mitochondrial energy production in the heart muscle. Here is the critical piece: statins deplete CoQ10. The drug they gave me to "protect" my heart was stripping away one of the molecules my heart needs most to function. When I was on statins, nobody told me to supplement CoQ10. Nobody mentioned that the drug was depleting my cardiac energy reserves while supposedly saving my life.

Magnesium Glycinate—300 to 400 mg before bed. Approximately 80 percent of the population is deficient. Supports heart rhythm, blood pressure, sleep, muscle recovery, and over 300 enzymatic reactions in the body. Glycinate is the most bioavailable form and does not cause digestive issues. Part of the Sinatra protocol alongside CoQ10.

Vitamin D3 with K2—I target a serum level of 60 to 80 ng/mL. Most people need 4,000 to 5,000 IU per day to reach that range. K2 ensures the calcium goes into your bones instead of your arteries. Always take with fat for absorption.

Omega-3 (EPA/DHA)—2 to 4 grams per day. High-quality fish oil or wild-caught fatty fish. Reduces triglycerides by 30 to 40 percent. Anti-inflammatory. Supports brain function and cardiovascular health.

Nattokinase and Lumbrokinase—These are natural fibrinolytic enzymes that support healthy blood flow and circulation. I take these instead of aspirin. Most cardiologists prescribe aspirin after a cardiac event. I chose evidence-based natural alternatives that support the same function without the gastrointestinal risks of long-term aspirin use.

A note on Niacin (Vitamin B3) and Lp(a)—I tried niacin to lower my genetically elevated Lp(a). It worked on the number. I brought it from 276 to 52. But my liver enzymes (AST and ALT) climbed, and my body told me to stop. So I stopped. I do not believe in artificially lowering a number my body produces for a reason. That is what statins do to LDL. I will not do the same thing to Lp(a). My approach now is to manage the root causes that make Lp(a) dangerous: insulin, inflammation, diet, and lifestyle. Fix the context. Respect the biology.

Armour Thyroid—125 mg. This is a natural thyroid supplement derived from porcine (pig) thyroid gland. It contains both T3 and T4, the actual thyroid hormones your body needs. Not the synthetic version that most doctors prescribe. My thyroid was flagged in four of seven panels over 14 years and nobody addressed it. When I finally did, this was the supplement that made the difference. It is the only thing I take that requires a prescription, and it is a natural gland extract, not a pharmaceutical drug.

That is the full protocol. Based on my blood work. Informed by Sinatra's research. Adjusted when my levels change. No aspirin. No statins. No pharmaceutical blood thinners.

> *For a supplement protocol based on your actual lab values, ask Neo at neo.healthtruth.ai*

I play competitive singles tennis with my 16-year-old son David. I keep up with him. At 58.

That is the proof that the protocol works. Not a gym selfie. Not a before-and-after photo. A father keeping up with his teenage son on a tennis court. The same sport that almost killed me six years ago.

What changed. I stopped thinking of exercise as a way to burn calories and started thinking of it as a way to maintain metabolic health. The shift is everything. When exercise is about calories, you eat garbage and try to outrun it. When exercise is about metabolic health, you move your body because it makes your insulin work better, your inflammation drop, your hormones function, and your brain stay sharp.

What I do. Tennis. Three to four times per week. Competitive singles. High-intensity interval work built into the sport naturally. Walking. Every day. Not on a treadmill. Outside. In the sun. Vitamin D production. Circadian rhythm. Stress reduction. All free. Resistance training. Bodyweight and weights. Not excessive. Enough to maintain muscle mass, which is one of the strongest predictors of longevity.

What I stopped doing. Long, grinding cardio sessions that I thought were "heart-healthy." Hours on the treadmill or the elliptical that were driving cortisol and inflammation without building the metabolic fitness that actually protects the heart. Exercising to eat. The old model: I worked out hard today so I can eat whatever I want tonight. That model almost killed me.

> *For a movement plan matched to your health profile and goals, ask Neo at neo.healthtruth.ai*

Sometimes what you stop doing matters more than what you start.

I stopped trusting one number. LDL cholesterol is a 1.4x risk factor. Diabetes is 10.71x. I stopped letting the weakest predictor on the list drive my entire treatment plan.

I stopped eating against my DNA. My APOE e4 genotype cannot process high-carbohydrate, low-fat diets without metabolic damage. I ate that diet for 30 years because the system told me to. I stopped.

I stopped ignoring my thyroid. Four flags in 14 years. Nobody mentioned it. I addressed it. It changed everything.

I stopped accepting "normal" as healthy. Standard lab ranges are built from a sick population. A fasting insulin of 24 is "normal." It is not healthy. A TSH of 4.5 is "normal." It is not optimal. I stopped accepting the ranges and started demanding functional optimal.

I stopped being afraid. This was the hardest one. The fear of dying consumed every breath for months after my heart attack. I stopped living in fear and started living in knowledge. I know my genetics. I know my markers. I know my risks. And I know what to do about them. Knowledge replaced fear. That is the real protocol.

If you do one thing after reading this book, do this.

Go to your doctor. Ask for fasting insulin and hs-CRP. Two tests. Under $60 combined. Available at any lab.

If your doctor says no, that tells you something. If your doctor says yes, the results will tell you everything.

A fasting insulin under 5 and an hs-CRP under 1.0 means your metabolic engine is running clean. You are not out of the woods forever, but you are in a very good place.

A fasting insulin above 8 or an hs-CRP above 2.0 means something is happening that your standard blood panel is not showing you. It means the root cause investigation needs to start. It means the 12-headed dragon might be waking up.

Two tests. Sixty dollars. The beginning of seeing clearly.

Or open Neo. Tap a button. And let the investigation begin.

neo.healthtruth.ai

The truth heals

ACKNOWLEDGMENTS

This book exists because of the people who believed in the truth before it was popular to tell it.

To Jane Ubell-Meyer and her company Bedside Reading, for her expertise in publishing and book marketing. Your guidance turned this story into a book the world can hold in its hands.

To Bill Ackman, for supporting the mission and the cause. Your conviction that the health system can be better gave me the confidence to build something that challenges it.

To the global metabolic health community, led by Prof. Tim Noakes, whose decades of courage in the face of institutional resistance paved the road that the rest of us now walk. You fought the fight before any of us knew there was a fight to be had.

Special thanks to Nina Teicholz, whose work changed how I understood food, fat, and the lies we were told. Your book gave me permission to eat the food that saved my life. Your friendship gave me the strength to write about it.

To Dr. Philip Ovadia, Dr. Aseem Malhotra, Dr. Robert Cywes, and Prof. Tim Noakes. You did not have to say yes. You said yes anyway. This platform and this book would not exist without your names, your science, and your willingness to stand behind a patient who refused to stay plugged in.

To Carl, Pat, Fred, and every person on those forums at 2 AM who shared their blood work, their stories, and their hope with a stranger. You saved my life. You did not know it at the time. But you did.

To my wife Melanie. The rock. The one who refused to let me drown. The one who said "you are going to make it" when I could not say it to myself.

To Sarah, Rebecca, and David. Everything I do is for you.

And to my father. Life is made up of moments and memories. This book is both.

ABOUT THE AUTHOR

MARK KAPLAN is the founder of HealthTruth | Neo, the first AI platform built on root cause science. He is a former ATP professional tennis player who competed at Wimbledon, played Pete Sampras at Queen's Club, and beat many former top 10 players including Patrick Rafter, a former world number 1. He was ranked number 117 ATP player in the world.

In 1989, Arthur Ashe presented Mark with the Division 1 college player of the year award at the US Open. Neither of them knew they shared the same genetic disease.

At 52, Mark had a heart attack on a tennis court despite being one of the fittest people in every room he walked into. Seven blood panels over 14 years had watched one number while eleven root causes went undetected. He fired his cardiologist, stopped the drugs, and spent six years investigating what went wrong. He reversed everything.

Today at 58, Mark is on zero medications with a metabolic age of 43. He plays competitive tennis with his 16-year-old son David, who carries the same genetic markers and was tested at 15. He built HealthTruth | Neo with four world-class doctors to ensure nobody else has to survive a heart attack before discovering the truth about their health.

Mark was born in Johannesburg, South Africa. He holds a BA in Economics and an MBA from UC Irvine. He lives in Stamford,

Connecticut with his wife Melanie and their three children, Sarah, Rebecca, and David.

> *He is not a doctor. He is a citizen scientist, a patient, and a heart attack survivor who believes the truth heals.*

CONTINUE THE JOURNEY

neo.healthtruth.ai
Scan to meet Neo. Ask your first question free.

Follow Mark on X: @markkaplan20

www.ingramcontent.com/pod-product-compliance
Lightning Source LLC
LaVergne TN
LVHW100315210926
848480LV00003B/1136